Tibetan Medicine Series
358EN

This volume contains the proceedings of the Tibetan Medicine Seminar held at the Convent of Santo Domingo and at the ULL (University of La Laguna), Pyramid Conference Hall, San Cristóbal de La Laguna, Tenerife, Spain January 11-17, 2013

Conference Organizers:

The International Dzogchen Community
The Shang Shung Institute, International Institute for Tibetan Studies
A.S.I.A., Association for International Solidarity in Asia
Arura Tibetan Medical Group

Sponsors:
San Cristóbal de La Laguna
ULL (Universidad de La Laguna)

Collaborators:

OCEANO Vitality Hotel & Medical Spa
Hacienda Cristóforo

Cover design by Yuchen Namkhai
Coordinated by Rita Bizzotto
English revision by Susan Schwarz

ISBN: 978-88-7834-146-3

2015, Shang Shung Edizioni
58031 Arcidosso - Italy
E-mail: shangshunged@tiscali.it
www.shangshungstore.org

TIBETAN MEDICINE SEMINAR

THIRD TIBETAN CULTURAL EVENT

On Birth, Life, and Death

CONVENT OF SANTO DOMINGO

SAN CRISTOBAL DE LA LAGUNA
TENERIFE - SPAIN

January 11-17, 2013

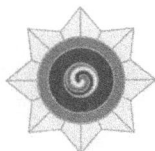

ཡེ་ཤེས་འཁོར་ལོ་ཚོགས་པི་ཡལ་འདེ་ས།

Shang Shung Publications

*This publication has been realized thanks to the
voluntary work of many people
from the International Dzogchen Community.*

*The printing expenses have been generously offered by
Chögyal Namkhai Norbu and Rosa Namkhai.*

Our heartfelt thanks go to them all.

Contents

Foreword

Tibetan medicine, an ancient profound knowledge, is slowly making headway, in the West, into the mainstream culture of health and well-being. This is thanks to the continuous, unrelenting efforts of many scholars and dedicated individuals and institutions. They tirelessly work to keep alive not only the medical tradition but also all aspects of Tibetan civilization with its rich, invaluable cultural heritage.

Among them is Chögyal Namkhai Norbu, a great scholar and Dzogchen Master, spiritual teacher of the Dzogchen Community, and founder of the Shang Shung Institute (International Institute for Tibetan Studies) and A.S.I.A. (Association for International Solidarity in Asia). Eminent Author of many groundbreaking works on Tibetan culture, medicine, and history (recent publications include *On Birth, Life and Death*; *Healing with Fire*; and the three-volume set *The Light of Kailash*), Chögyal Namkhai Norbu has dedicated his entire life to preserving and making available to the general public the precious treasure of the Tibetan culture, which in our era faces unprecedented challenges to its very survival. It is vitally important to make accessible, through diverse tools of communication and through concrete projects, this vast body of knowledge, permitting as many as possible to benefit from it. It is equally important to keep this knowledge alive in its motherland, its irreplaceable source and soul, Tibet.

For this reason during the Third Tibetan Cultural Event, held in Tenerife (Spain) in 2013, focusing mainly on Tibetan medicine, and in the presence of distinguished Tibetan doctors residing and working both in Tibet and in the West, a collaborative agreement was signed by Shang Shung Institute and Arura, a Tibetan medical association based in

Tibet, in an area traditionally known as Amdo. Arura is one of the largest Tibetan medical organizations in the world with five major institutions. The Arura President graciously presented to Chögyal Namkhai Norbu a multi-volume (60-volume set) encyclopedia of the medical traditions in Tibet, a work of immense value and interest and one of Arura's most important projects.

The possibility of the East and West working together, sharing and integrating different bodies of knowledge, while respecting and holding in high estimation each other's differences will not only help to keep the Tibetan culture alive but also enrich Western culture and the lives of countless people.

Fabio Andrico

Brief Biographies of the Speakers

Professor Namkhai Norbu

Namkhai Norbu, one of the foremost living Dzogchen masters, was born in Derge, East Tibet, in 1938. While still very young he was sent to important Buddhist monasteries and colleges where he completed the rigorous traditional study program, the Five Major Arts (Literature, Medicine, Philosophy, Astrology, History), and the Five Minor Arts, acquiring vast and profound knowledge and receiving degrees in Tibetan Medicine and Philosophy and Literature.

In 1955, he met Rigdzin Changchub Dorje (1826-1961), his principal Dzogchen teacher, whose lifestyle and way of teaching inspired him profoundly. Invited by the Chinese authorities, from 1954 to 1957 he was instructor of Tibetan language at the Southwestern University for the Minorities in Cheng-tu (Sze Chuang), People's Republic of China, and thus he had the opportunity to learn classical Chinese and Mongolian languages.

In 1958 he was in India for a pilgrimage and, on account of the serious political events in his own country, he was not able to return in Tibet. In India he spent two years as author and chief editor of Tibetan textbooks at the Development Office of the Government of Sikkim, in the town of Gangtok. In 1960 Professor Namkhai Norbu started his academic collaboration with Prof. Tucci at ISMEO (Istituto per il Medio e Estremo Oriente – Institute of the Middle and Far East) in Rome, Italy.

From 1962 to 1992 he taught Tibetan and Mongolian Language and Literature at the Istituto Universitario Orientale di Napoli (University of Oriental Studies in Naples). In addition to his activities all over the world as a spiritual master, Namkhai Norbu focused his thirty years of research mainly on the ancient history of Tibet, thoroughly investigating the autochthonous pre-Buddhist Bön tradition and the monarchic age connected to the Shang Shung kingdom.

Other fields of his research were the origin, theory, and practice of astrology and, above all, Tibetan traditional medicine, a medical system that integrates the highest aspects of the culture's science and spirituality into a comprehensive system of health and healing. He also deeply studied the Tibetan nomad civilization. Among the books he wrote on these subjects are: *A Journey into the Culture of Tibetan Nomads*; *Drung Deu Bön*; *The Necklace of Zhi*; *Zhang Zhung: Images from a Lost Kingdom*; *The Light of Kailash* (3 volumes); *Healing with Fire: A Practical Manual of Tibetan Moxibustion*; *The Practice of Tibetan Kunye Massage*; *Yantra Yoga: The Tibetan Yoga of Movement*; *On Birth, Life and Death*; and *Tibetan Yoga of Movement: The Art and Practice of Yantra Yoga*. Towards the end of the 1980s, Chögyal Namkhai Norbu founded ASIA (Association for International Solidarity in Asia), an NGO committed to cooperation and development not only in Asia but all over the world, and ISSI (International Shang Shung Institute), which works to preserve and divulge Tibetan culture in the West.

Dr. O Tsokchen (Ai Cuo Qian)

Dr. O Tsokchen holds a medical (M.D.) degree in Biomedicine and is one of the leading experts on Tibetan medicine today. Currently, Dr. Tsokchen is Professor and the President of Tso-ngon (Qinghai) University Tibetan Medical College, as well as President of Tso-ngon Provincial Tibetan Medical Hospital and Director of the P. R. China National Museum of Tibetan Medicine. Additionally, Dr. Tsokchen holds the position of President of Tso-ngon Tibetan Medicine Association and Honorary President of Tso-ngon Biomedical College of Tso-ngon University.

With these responsibilities and under his leadership, Dr. Tsokchen has worked tirelessly with his Tibetan medicine teams at these institutions to establish, improve, and develop Tibetan medical teachings, clinical practices, and research since the1980s, mainly in Tso-ngon Province of P.R. China. Dr. Tsokchen established an academic training system of Tibetan medicine including bachelor, master, and doctoral levels in clinical medicine, pharmaceuticals, and Tibetan medicine managementat Tso-ngon University Tibetan Medical College. Many of the students who have graduated under Tso-ngon University Tibetan Medical College are now working at the provincial, prefectural, county, and township levels of prominent health facilities.

Tso-ngon Provincial Tibetan Medical Hospital is one of the leading Tibetan medical hospitals in Tibetan regions today, and under Dr. Tsokchen's guidance and management it has evolved into the national standard facility for Tibetan hospitals. Dr. Tsokchen also founded Arura Tibetan Medicine Group, which produces more than three hundred kinds of medicine for clinical treatment. Many of the medicines are used in cities and regions throughout China. Furthermore, in the interest of preserving and promoting Tibetan medicine practices, Dr. Tsokchen has established the P.R. China National Museum of Tibetan Medicine, where he leads a team of colleagues to collect historic Tibetan medicine books and publish these rare treasures. To date the museum has published more than one hundred old Tibetan medicine books and some forty national university level Tibetan medicine textbooks, which are the main teaching textbooks used in most of the Tibetan medical institutions in Tibetan areas.

With the development of modern science, Tibetan medicine is required to perform its clinical treatments and medicine scientifically; for this reason, Dr. Tsokchen established the Tso-ngon (Qinghai) Provincial Research Institution of Tibetan Medicine where studies are conducted as clinical trials to test Tibetan medicine and its treatments. Several of these same studies were selected and awarded as "best research" at the provincial level in 2001 and 2004. In addition, Dr. Tsokchen has co-authored and edited ten books and numerous articles on Tibetan medical theory, the production of Tibetan medicine, and its various treatments.

Dr. Lhusham Gyal

Dr. Lhusham Gyal is Professor and Dean of Tso Ngon (Qinghai) University Tibetan Medical College in Siling (Xining), P.R. China. He received his Tibetan medicine training with many Tibetan senior teachers throughout the Tibetan regions, including Amdo and U-tsang, and obtained his bachelor and master degrees in Medical Studies from Tibet University, Tibetan Autonomous Region.

Dr. Lhusham Gyal is one of the best-known young Tibetan medical doctors inside of Tibet today. In particular, he is recognized as the author of *A Systemic Analysis of Tibetan Medical Psychology*, the first book of its kind anywhere, published by the Beijing National Publishing House in 2004, for which he has received several awards, both locally and internationally. Dr. Gyal is also the author of numerous articles and books, and associate editor-in-chief of the textbook series *Curricula of National Tibetan Medical Majors in University*.

Dr. Gyal's work as a professor, physician, and author has inspired many throughout Tibet and China, and beyond: he has been awarded many honors such as "Excellent Teacher" by both Qinghai Province and Trace Foundation (in New York City).

Dr. Kunchok Gyaltsen

Dr. Kunchok Gyaltsen, a Tibetan medical doctor and Buddhist monk, is one of a new generation of outstanding Tibetan medical doctors. Having spent his life gaining expertise in both Tibetan Buddhist studies and Tibetan medicine, Dr. Gyaltsen's proficiency in clinical treatment (specializing in digestive disorders), his many public teachings and scholarly writings on the approaches of Tibetan medicine, combined with twenty-five years of training as a Tibetan Buddhist monk, make him exceptionally knowledgeable in ways to keep the body, mind, and spirit healthy.

Dr. Kunchok Gyaltsen is an honorary Associate Professor at Qinghai University Tibetan Medical College; assistant editor and translator (Chinese to Tibetan) of a medical textbook on western epidemiology, part of a twenty-eight book series for university medical courses for Tibetans; and the coauthor of a medical textbook on diagnosis, part of a Tibetan medical textbook series entitled *21st Century Medical College Textbook Series (2005)*.

In 2001, Dr. Gyaltsen founded the Tibetan Healing Fund, a nonprofit organization with offices in both Qinghai Province (Amdo), P.R. China, and Seattle, Washington, whose mission is to provide basic education and primary health care to rural Tibetan women and children. Today the Tibetan Healing Fund serves a growing number of isolated and impoverished women and children in the Tibetan regions of northwestern P.R. China. Tibetan Healing Fund projects include bilingual and bicultural education, community midwife training, health education and outreach, and building the first Tibetan natural birth and health-training center.

Dr. Gyaltsen holds a Ph.D. in Public Health from UCLA, where he was a recipient of the Fred H. Bixby Doctoral Fellowship. Dr. Gyaltsen also holds two master degrees, one in Primary Healthcare Management from ASEAN Institute for Health Development at Mahidol University, Bangkok, Thailand, and another in International and Intercultural Management from the School for International Training in Vermont. Dr. Gyaltsen has conducted significant public health research in Thailand, Burma, Nepal, Laos, and P.R. China.

Dr. Phuntsog Wangmo

Menpa (doctor) Phuntsog Wangmo received her advanced degree from the Lhasa University School of Traditional Medicine in 1988 where she also served a two-year residency after completing her five-year training program (1983-1990). During that time she studied with the *khenpos* Troru Tsenam and Gyaltsen, two of Tibet's foremost doctors who are credited with the revival of Tibetan medicine within Tibet under the Chinese. Dr. Phuntsog Wangmo had the exceptional opportunity of extensive clinical training under Khenpo Troru Tsenam for four years. Thereafter, she dedicated many years of work as a doctor in Eastern Tibet, where she collaborated and directed the implementation of A.S.I.A., the nonprofit organization founded by Chögyal Namkhai Norbu. Since that time, she has worked on behalf of A.S.I.A. setting up hospitals and training centers in the remote regions of Sichuan Province and Chamdo Perfecture.

From 1996 to present, she has been the A.S.I.A. project coordinator in Tibet for the development of Gamthog Hospital in collaboration with expatriate personnel as well as the overall health coordinator and practitioner of traditional Tibetan medicine supervising health activities throughout the surrounding region of Chamdo Perfecture. Prior to 1996, she was on the faculty of Shang Shung Institute in Italy where she gave numerous seminars and conference presentations on Tibetan medicine. Dr. Wangmo is based at the Shang Shung Institute of America where she is the director of the Institute's Traditional Tibetan Medicine Program.

Fabio Andrico

Born and raised in Italy, Fabio Andrico is an internationally recognized expert on Yantra Yoga. Graduate in Oriental Studies at the Oriental University Institute of Naples, Italy, he is one of the closest students of the great Dzogchen master Chögyal Namkhai Norbu, who introduced Yantra Yoga to the West in the early 1970s.

Andrico, who initially studied Hatha Yoga in India, has been learning, practicing, teaching, and writing about Yantra Yoga since the late 1970s. He regularly conducts courses, workshops, and teacher trainings around the world, and has appeared in yoga DVDs such as *The Eight Movements of Yantra Yoga*; *Breathe*; and *Tibetan Yoga of Movement: Perfect Rhythm of Life*, Levels 1 and 2. He coauthored *Tibetan Yoga of Movement: The Art and Practice of Yantra Yoga* with Chögyal Namkhai Norbu and also collaborated on the book *Yantra Yoga: The Tibetan Yoga of Movement*.

Aldo Oneto

Aldo Oneto is director of Shang Shung Institute in Italy. As a practitioner of reflexology for more than twenty years, after studying the three-year course at the International Shang Shung Institute in Milan and at Merigar, Tuscany, he gained a qualification in Tibetan Kunye Massage. Later, he underwent another two-year in-depth instructors program and is now one of the principal Kunye instructors for the Institute. He has been teaching courses for several years internationally.

PRESENTATION

NAMKHAI NORBU:

Origin and History of Tibetan Medicine

January 11, evening

I want to say something before we start the conference. I am sorry I do not speak the Spanish language well, but we have translators so you can understand. We are in webcast so I need to start.

Good evening everyone and everywhere. Here we are in Tenerife, starting today our programs of Tibetan culture. This year they are especially dedicated to the medical field. You will have the occasion to learn something; this is really a good opportunity. In these days we have distinguished medical professionals guests from Tibet so I will not talk about medicine.

Instead, I would like to explain a little about the background of Tibetan culture, because this may be useful to understand why it is important to learn a little about the various fields it includes, such as history, medicine, astrology, and so on. As you all know Tibet is called the Land of Snows and also the roof of the world because it is situated in the Himalayas. This has created a special condition: while, on the one hand, its isolation has not favored material development as has happened in other countries, on the other hand it has allowed ancient culture and knowledge to remain intact and be handed down over the centuries.

Let me give you the example of the Buddhist tradition. Buddhism, all the teachings of Sutra and Tantra, were developed in India and in the country of Oddiyana. Already in ancient times the Tibetans showed great interest in the spiritual path. Since development and communications at the physical level were not very easy, they dedicated themselves more to the spiritual path, which was of course very developed, just like in India and Oddiyana. Many Tibetan scholars made sacrifices to go to India and Oddiyana to study and translate the ancient texts and to invite to Tibet important masters who developed and enriched the spirituality of Tibet. Today, if we consider ancient cultures and knowledge, the richest spiritual path is in Tibet, also thanks to its geographic isolation.

When we organize an event about Tibetan culture many people might think that we are doing it because Namkhai Norbu is Tibetan and likes his culture, but it is not the only reason. Tibetan culture has great value for the whole world, not only for the Tibetans. It is important that people understand this. That is why last year we organized a ten-day cultural event on Tibet and we were very pleased with the enthusiastic participation of people and the fact that the local authorities worked with us in the organization. This is something important for all of us citizens of the world.

In general, official history traces the culture and knowledge of India and China back four thousand years and we consider this very ancient time. But the history and the culture of Tibet also date from the same period. I worked for nearly thirty years at the University and in the last years I dedicated myself particularly to research on Tibetan culture and history and found out that they are very old, almost as old as Indian and Chinese. For example, the Buddhist tradition is widespread in Tibet, but before this there was a pre-Buddhist tradition, a kind of religion called Bön. How did it develop? We consider that its founder was Tonpa Shenrab, and we find explanations of the Bön tradition from him. From here we can understand how Tibetan culture developed originally.

The majority of Western scholars follow the Tibetan Buddhist tradition, the way that history is presented by Buddhism. But this does not reflect the real situation of Tibet. To know about the history of ancient Tibet we have to go into the field of the Bön tradition because Buddhism began much later, with the generations of the Tibetan kings. According to the history of the Bön tradition, before the famous king Songtsen Gampo there were thirty-two generations of Tibetan kings. Traditionally it is considered that the origin of Tibetan history coincides with the coronation of the first Tibetan king, but this is not so, it is much earlier, around the time of the famous "Miu dung trug," the story of six brothers, which is considered to be the origin of the Tibetans and which both the ancient tradition and the Buddhist agree upon. But where were these six brothers from? The Buddhist interpretation is different from that of the ancient Bön tradition. The latter, for example, presents the origin of humanity as the cosmic egg. Some scholars believe that this tradition is Hindu, but the fact that this explanation exists in Hindu Shaivism does not imply that it has originated in Hinduism. Why? The Shaivas consider that the most important sacred place is Mount Kailash. Even today many of them make sacrifices to go to Tibet to visit and circumambulate it. Therefore Shaivism does not come first but rather Kailash. And Kailash is in Tibet, not in India. So when they speak of the cosmic egg, there is no contradiction.

"Cosmic Egg" is how the five elements are put together and how countries, beings, and so on developed from these. This is explained in the ancient Bön tradition. When I started doing this kind of research I wrote a book called *The Necklace of Jewels* (*Norbu Doshal*), which is published in India. In it I explained very clearly what it meant by cosmic egg and that there is no contradiction. In the ancient Bön tradition it says that all beings came from the cosmic egg, that human beings developed from the three original groups of gods, *nagas*, and *nyen*. *The Unique Volume of the Lang Clan* (*Rlangs kyi po ti bse ru rgyas pa*), a very ancient history of Tibet, explains the origin of human beings, and in particular the Tibetans, with the cosmic egg and six brothers from whom the six Tibetan tribes originated. Among these, two had particular significance for the history of Tibet: one tribe prospered and ruled western Tibet, which is the region called Shang Shung, while the other scattered in eastern Tibet. The first tribe, named Khyung, had more advanced understanding because as the Bön tradition affirms, the famous Bön teacher Tönpa Shenrab created the Shang Shung writing, which did not exist previously. Therefore, the history of Shang Shung also began from the time of Tönpa Shenrab, while, at the time, Tibet did not exist yet. The other tribes of the six brothers, for example, were very strong physically and they had a history, but writing only developed in Western Tibet. Therefore, to study the origin of Tibetan history and culture we must go back to that.

In Tibet, in general, the most widespread tradition states that Tibetan writing developed in the time of Songtsen Gampo and that before him there was none. This is true, there was no Tibetan writing, but it does not mean that the Tibetans did not *use* a form of writing, they used that of Shang Shung. When Songtsen Gampo wanted to create a Tibetan culture and knowledge, he said Tibetans needed Tibetan writing, which meant *not* the Shang Shung writing. Why did he say this? There are very specific reasons. When the lineage of the Tibetan kings began – Nyatri Tsenpo was the first – for five or six generations they all ruled by following and using the language and culture of Shang Shung because Shang Shung was the origin of the Bön tradition, which at that time was considered a religion. Of course it was not similar to Buddhism, it was very different, and I will give you an example.

When we speak of the elements – earth, water, fire, and air – the ancient Bön tradition did not present them as they do now. Today there is a modern Bön tradition that presents them more or less as in Buddhism because it has assimilated everything from the Buddhist tradition and has developed a modern form of Bön. But when we speak of the ancient Bön we have to understand their original way of seeing. In Tibet we have prayer flags: in the corners are four animals and at the center is a horse, hence their name, *lungta* or wind horse. But what do these four animals represent? When we talk about the five elements, or the four active elements, the ancient Bön tradition presents something that has life in the dimension of the element, with animals such as the tiger, the lion, the dragon, and the eagle.

The eagle is very important in the ancient Bön tradition, which is the only one to represent a deity or a potential, something superior, which is always symbolized by a fire eagle. Fire is the symbol of energy and is material, but has a potential, a power, a function. This function is alive and moves, and is represented by the eagle.

Then the dragon, *chusin*. It is considered to be a mythical water animal, so it remains in the dimension of water. In this way not only is the material aspect of water presented, but the dimension with life, movement, and energy.

The lion represents the earth element. How can we understand this? For example, the Tibetans, just like the Chinese, believe that there are snow lions – it can also be a legend, but in any case we have this concept. Snow is found in the high mountains, such as Mount Everest, which are a mixture of earth and rock. It is a concentration of the substance of the earth element and in this dimension there is a being that has life. This being is the lion.

Then the tiger: in general we find the tiger in the forest, where there is a lot of wood. In the astrological system, both in the Chinese and Tibetan tradition, the air element is represented by wood. Wood means trees and in the forest the animal that represents this movement is the tiger.

In the Buddhist tradition the elements are not presented in this way so why do we have these figures in the Buddhist *lungta*? Because the Buddhist tradition evolved from India to Tibet. Firstly, the Tibetan king invited Shantarakshita, a famous master who gave teachings from the Buddhist tradition. But he did not manage to spread them because for centuries the Tibetans had followed the Bön tradition and found too much difference between the two. For this reason Shantarakshita eventually returned to India and advised the king to invite Guru Padmasambhava, a great tantric practitioner who possessed high knowledge of the level of energy.

When Guru Padmasambhava came to Tibet, since he knew about the attitude of the people, their beliefs and their desires, he communicated the *essence* of the Buddhist teaching and not the outward aspect of applying it. The Tibetans were used to following the ancient Bön tradition and he retained it, but by combining the essence of Buddhism with their practices. For this reason, the Buddhism of Tibet is often called Lamaism, because it has different characteristics as Guru Padmasambhava integrated many aspects of the Bön tradition.

I will give another example. On important days such as the anniversary of the birth of the Dalai Lama, or when we have to carry out important activities, we always do the Sang ritual. The meaning of this ritual is to purify our dimension and also ourselves through the smoke by burning aromatic herbs. For Tibetans Sang is important but this ritual actually comes from the ancient Bön tradition. We can understand this from the fact that at the beginning of the rite of Sang called *gyagnen*, which is now diffused in all traditions, there is an explanation of its origin, a tradition that belonged to ancient Bön and is not found in Buddhism. This tradition is called *chorab*. Sometimes it is also called *mang*, meaning there is something more connected with the energy level. I worked a lot on this, reading many ancient books, but I could find no explanations. Finally I discovered that in the rites, the simple rituals used in the countryside, there is a so-called *chorab* explaining their history. Then I made a collection of these types of rituals and studied all *chorabs* in order to reconstruct their history. For example, the rite of Sang called *gyagnen* is a word of Guru Padmasambhava. At the beginning it says "Father Sky and Mother Land" (and between them there is all the Atmosphere, which is our condition). In the Buddhist tradition this kind of expression had never been used, this belongs to the ancient Bön tradition. But Guru Padmasambhava was going into essence and did not limit only to words. When you do research, you have to be totally free and have no preconceptions. You should not have a limited point of view and think that everything must correspond to your own tradition. This is how you can find the real condition. I have carried out research on ancient Tibetan history in this way. This work resulted in three volumes on the period from the birth of Tönpa Shenrab to the present that have been published for many years in China. The first two volumes are now also available in English translation. So I understood that this year is 3929, starting from the year of birth of Tonpa Shenrab. Why? Because astrology, the way it is presented in the Bön tradition, started with that date.

For this reason I believe that the culture and history of Tibet are of great value and are just as ancient as those of India and China. When I started my work at the university at first I was very surprised because all the professors believed that the history and culture of Tibet began from the time of Songtsen Gampo. I thought it could not be, but this was the official view. Early in my research I found it very difficult because I could not find evidence of a culture or a writing dating back to before the time that the Buddhist tradition arrived in Tibet. I could only deduce it with logic. But gradually as I went ahead with my research I found concrete evidence.

For example, the last Shang Shung king was killed by Songtsen Gampo and, from that time, the kingdom of Shang Shung passed under Tibet. Before Songtsen Gampo, many Tibetan kings (such as, for example, the famous king Trigum Tsenpo, who was against the Bön tradition) had tried to take possession of Shang Shung, which was a great and powerful kingdom, but they had never succeeded because Tibet was not under a single Tibetan king, but divided into several tribes. In addition, the Tibetan kings and kingdoms followed the Bön tradition and culture of Shang Shung so Tibet was totally dependent. Songtsen Gampo, however, was a very intelligent king and knew very well that Shang Shung was stronger than Tibet and so he adopted a policy of alliances through marriage. He made his sister marry the king of the Shang Shung and he himself married a princess of Shang Shung, thus creating a very close relationship. He also understood that if Tibet did not have knowledge and a culture of its own, independent of Shang Shung, it would never become strong. So he also took a queen from Nepal and from China and strove to introduce into Tibet not only the Buddhist tradition, but also culture and knowledge. He sent one of his ministers, Thönmi Sambhota, to India to study and create a Tibetan form of writing. In my opinion, this was only possible thanks to the fact that Tibetans were already using a writing, that of Shang Shung, and it could not have taken place if they had been, as some scholars state, totally devoid of writing and culture. This theory is also supported by logic.

The writing of Shang Shung and the Tibetan writing created by Thönmi Sambhota are not the same thing and in my history book I have explained this very well. For example, in Tibet we have two types of writing, *uchen* and *umed*. *Uchen* is the Indian style letters created by Thönmi Sambhota who also created the grammatical system from Sanskrit. In Tibetan, we write in *umed* which I believe originates from the writing of the Shang Shung. For example, if we write a letter of the alphabet using the language of Thönmi Sambhota, we start from the top of the letter and write from left to right, then we complete the letter. If, on the other hand, we write in *umed,* we write from right to left, so we can write very quickly. A leading scholar who did research on Tibetan history said that when we write in *uchen* quickly it becomes *umed*. It is impossible. I always agree on what he says, but I do not agree on this point.

A good example is Bhutan. In Bhutan there is a script called *gyuyig*, which I know very well. *Gyuyig* is *uchen*. For centuries they have written it very quickly and it has become *gyuyig*, but it is always written from left to right. Even if they write it quickly, it will never become *umed*. Therefore I am very convinced that the source of *umed* is Shang Shung. There are two or three different scripts that come from Shang Shung, such as *marchen* and *marchung.* In the language of Shang Shung *mar* means divinity. When I was in Tibet I had the good fortune to learn from a famous Tibetan writer a form of writing called *lhabab yige*: *lha* means divinity, *bab* means that it comes from there. In the language of Shang Shung, this corresponds to *mar*, divinity. Later I realized that this is the origin of Tibetan *umed*. I learned these letters and I wrote them for myself, no one knew this writing. After three months, the teacher who had taught me died.

More than two years later in Jeykundo, I met a very special Tibetan doctor who had gone to India many times and knew many things. In his room I saw some verses he had written in *lhabab yige*. I looked at them and read them. They were four verses from the *Bodhisattvacaryavatara* of Shantideva that say: "All happiness comes from the desire to benefit others; all suffering comes from the wish for happiness for ourselves." When I read these verses in *lhabab yige* the doctor was very surprised that I knew this writing and asked me from where I had learned it. I told him that I learnt it from a calligrapher who also wrote the Kangyur in gold, in the time when there was the king of Derge. I then asked him if he knew its origin, and he replied that he did not know, but that it was called *lhabab yige*. This is an example of the origin of Tibetan writing.

So in Tibet the Shang Shung writing was used. And there was not only the knowledge from Bön but also a lot of knowledge and understanding. For example, Tibetan medicine, astrology, and many types of arts all originally existed in Shang Shung and we can understand this from the books that come from the Tunhuang documents.

The Tunhuang documents, an important collection of ancient books written in Chinese and Tibetan that date back to the period of the last kings of Tibet, are considered very important for Chinese, Tibetan, and Western scholars. They remained under the sand for many centuries. When they reappeared many scholars and professors, particularly English and French, took them to their countries. Today many of them are found in museums in London and Paris and are very important also for research into Tibetan history. I myself went to Kansu Province, near Qinghai, to visit Tunhuang, and when I do research I always use them a lot. For example, the information about the politics of marriages of Songtsen Gampo that I was telling before comes from that source. Based on these documents I have written a book entitled *Drung Deu Bön: Narrations, Symbolic Languages and the Bön Tradition in Ancient Tibet*, which contains some very interesting explanations. What we mean by "ancient Bön tradition" can be found there. And at the time of the

Tibetan kings there were twelve different kinds of Bön traditions. In this way they were developed in Tibet.

When we speak about Tibetan medicine most people think that it comes from the Indian Ayurvedic tradition. Of course it developed from India, China, and different countries, but medicine and astrology already existed in Shang Shung. In fact, among the Tunhuang documents there are two authentic texts on medicine. Therefore Tibetan medicine comes from Shang Shung, and it is important to know this. So Tibetan culture has value, knowledge, and understanding that is very rich. Many Westerners, for example, think that the spiritual path of Buddhism is very developed in Tibet. This is true, but there is not only this aspect. Tibet is a highly important source for many aspects of knowledge, and thus a precious treasure for all humanity and not just for Tibetans. It is very important that we learn and translate and understand, so that it becomes alive. That is why we are working also on that field. If there is a valid profound culture and knowledge and we do not discover it and do not spread and lose it, we lose something very precious. If we understand it, if we study it, if we use it, we will all be enriched in our knowledge, values, and humanity. For this it is important to know and to keep alive Tibet's cultural and spiritual heritage.

For example, since today many people are interested in spirituality I work with them and help them to understand. And the spiritual path I am teaching – which is called Dzogchen – is now very diffused. Generally people think of Buddhism as the teaching of Buddha Shakyamuni, but in Buddhism there are many different types of knowledge, many kinds of teachings and traditions. The Dzogchen teaching has developed and continued in the Buddhist tradition in Tibet for centuries. But it did not only start with Buddha Shakyamuni, it is one of the most ancient teachings that exist. When we explain about the Dzogchen teaching we speak about the twelve primordial masters. They lived in twelve different epochs. The first, Tönpa Nangwa Tampa, taught in a very ancient time, the Kalpa Dzogden, in which human beings were like *deva*s, gods, just as they are presented, for example, in the ancient tradition of India.

The Dzogchen teaching is not a tradition or a religion or a philosophy: the real sense of Dzogchen is beyond these definitions. It is knowledge, it is understanding, it is discovering the true nature of the individual who normally does not know it. With the Dzogchen teaching first of all we discover it and then we have to find ourselves in that state. This is what I teach in general.

This precious teaching has been preserved and continued in Tibet. If there were no Tibetans, if it were not for their knowledge and culture, it would no longer exist. For this reason it is also important to know the background of the history and culture of Tibet.

At the time of the famous king Songtsen Gampo, who also introduced the Buddhist tradition in Tibet, and of Trisong Detsen, who invited Guru Padmasambhava, many medical experts were invited not only from Tibet but from various different countries, and thus knowledge of medicine became very extensive. You see, today we have received all these volumes, they are more than sixty: they are not copies of a single book; it is a collection of all Tibetan medicine books in Tibet. So you can understand how developed Tibetan medicine is. Originally, when we speak about early Tibetan medicine we refer to the famous Four Tantras, and when we study we focus primarily on these. But of course, not only these Four Tantras exist; there are also many other different aspects of treatment, study, and learning. Some people consider it important to discuss whether they were originally introduced from India. I do not think that this is the key point, but rather that a great deal of knowledge has been accrued in Tibetan medicine.

We also have various aspects of astrology, which is also part of medicine. The Bön master Tönpa Shenrab taught all his knowledge to his second son, Chebu Trishe (Chebu means someone experienced in all therapies) who became a very important source for Tibetan medicine. We also know about *juthig*, a type of divination, from him. Tibetan medicine, in fact, has important characteristics that are different from Western. From the beginning, when we examine a person, we have to determine whether his illness is due to a negative provocation (*dönche*) or not (*dönmed*). If it is not only a physical illness and there is a negative provocation, an ordinary doctor is not sufficient and the patient should contact a doctor with spiritual knowledge and understanding. To find out, there is also *juthig*, a type of divination, a very ancient form of knowledge that has come from Shang Shung and still exists today. Ju Mipham, a famous and fairly recent Nyingmapa scholar, claimed to have read thirteen volumes of *juthig* in the Bön tradition and to have written the essence of them in a large volume that we still have today. Studying the *juthig* to understand how to do it is quite complicated. Today, even in the Bön tradition, there are no longer thirteen volumes, but only four or five. Many of those mentioned by Ju Mipham are gone and I was unable to find them.

When I returned to China, to Tibet, for the first time in 1982, in Lhasa I met an old Bönpo who came from Kongpo. In Kongpo there is a sacred mountain called Kongpo Bonri, and he had spent many years there. He had heard that Namkhai Norbu was doing research on Bön, and that he would like to hear something about it, so he came to visit me. He was not a scholar and knew nothing about history. He was a native of the Bön tradition and only knew how to perform some rituals. He told me that he had three books: one was a volume on *juthig*, another was on Shang Shung Meri, a deity of the ancient Bön tradition – they were building a kind of temple dedicated to this deity for producing their potentiality or power, called Shang Shung Chogkhar, and he had a book about how to build the Chogkhar. The third book explained about the sacred places of Kongpo Bönri. He told me that during the Cultural Revolution he had kept these books secretly and still had them. I asked him if he could show them to me. The book about *juthig* was a very large volume, while the others were smaller, about thirty pages. I asked him if I could photograph them and he gave me permission.

Later I took them to Italy and the text of the Shang Shung Meri Chogkhar became very important for my research (I found a copy of it also in Professor Tucci's library, some words just a little different). It is really interesting. In fact, when I made a trip to the USA, I went to

Arizona to visit the Indians. They showed me the *kivas* that date back to their ancient traditions: they were built underground, but they did not know exactly how they had been built because they had all been destroyed; only ruins of the flooring remained. Watching them, I realized that these bases were exactly the same as the Shang Shung Chogkhar. I was really surprised that the traditions of Shang Shung had a connection with the Indians of Arizona. Clearly it is a very ancient connection, perhaps even before the lands of the earth parted and became separate countries. Anyway it proved very useful and made me understand many things about the ancient Bön tradition.

In addition to divination, astrology also existed in ancient Shang Shung. In Tibet, in particular, we have two astrological systems, the Kartsi and the Nagtsi. The former is also widespread in the West and is the zodiac system, while the Nagtsi is based on the elements and connected to the lunar calendar. In Tibet, many people believe that it comes from China, because the word *gya* is often mentioned and many scholars consider that Gya is China. However, in the Bön tradition there are abundant explanations that Gya is not China but rather Shang Shung Phugpa, located in Inner Shang Shung. And there are all the explanations of the origin of the arts, of how to build stupas, temples etc. Therefore, many sources of Tibetan culture and knowledge are linked to Shang Shung. Many years ago when I began to speak about Shang Shung and to hold seminars explaining how the history of Shang Shung was linked to the Tibetan culture most of our professors at the university were laughing at me, they thought it was my fantasy. At that time nobody was speaking about Shang Shung, but today all scholars cannot disregard it.

With regard to the writing of Shang Shung, I said that at first I could not find concrete evidence of its existence. Eventually I came to know about the seal of the last king of Shang Shung that had been found in Menri in central Tibet. Menri was a very important Bön monastery, mentioned in the Tunhuang documents. When Songtsen Gampo killed the last king of Shang Shung, the Bönpo directed their black magic against him and he was struck by a serious illness that no one could cure. From the earliest kings up to the last one called Langdarma, there had always been two Bönpo masters among the royal masters. Even Trisong Detsen, who was a very Buddhist king, traditionally had to have two Bön masters among his own. When a prince was born it was they who did the purification ritual or the *trü*. Even the name of the king had to be given by the Bön masters and not the Buddhist, and for this reason most of the Buddhist kings had names in the Shang Shung language such as Agsho Leg, Thisho Leg, Desho Leg, and so on. Why did they keep this tradition? One of the reasons was not to receive the black magic of the Bön.

When Songtsen Gampo was struck by this serious illness, his Bönpo masters advised him to invite one of the most famous and powerful Shang Shung Bönpo masters of the period, Nangzher Löpo, who had sent him the magic power, otherwise he would never be healed. Nangzher Löpo came to Tibet, performed various rituals and Songtsen Gampo overcame his illness. To thank him the king gave him some land where today there is still the Bön institution of Menri. Nangzher Löpo brought the seal of the last king of Shang Shung there, where some of the objects of the Shang Shung kings are also preserved. This seal has now arrived in India, at the Bönpo Thobgyal Sarpa center. The seal is very large and contains an inscription in the language of Shang Shung: *Shang shung sipai gyalpo*, that is, the All-Conquering Universal King. This shows that there was a Shang Shung writing, as is also confirmed in the Bön tradition.

Some years ago, some Chinese scholars went to western Tibet and found examples of Shang Shung writing – an article appeared in a major Chinese newspaper – thus confirming that it existed. In addition, the kingdom of Shang Shung also extended into Ladakh and Lahaul, areas that are currently part of India. Here, too, we can find traces of the Shang Shung language, for example, in the dialects of certain areas. Years ago a sort of tablet with writing on it was found in the ground. Indian scholars thought it was the writing of some ethnic group from

India, but in the end British scholars discovered that it was the language of Shang Shung. So, you see, today nobody doubts any longer the existence of Shang Shung writing. This is something very important for the background of Tibetan history and culture.

Tibetan medicine is another patrimony for humanity. It did not develop only at the physical, material level, such as Western medicine, but considers the person as a whole of body, energy, and mind. As I have already said, in a diagnosis from the beginning you have to check whether there are negative provocations or not. It is easier to identify negative provocations in their material aspect. But there are also many aspects relating to energy and that, usually, we call black magic. In general we ignore how our dimension, our situation, is.

For example, when we say that there are spirits, local guardians, and so on, many people say they do not believe it because they have never seen them. That is not logical, and this is also confirmed by a very high level scholar in the Sakyapa tradition, Sakyapandita. You cannot see the past or the future, but you cannot deny them. You cannot see something that is far away. Science explains that it takes light many years to get to us. We cannot see where it comes from, but if we look at the night sky we can see how many stars there are. We know that the stars are constellations, solar systems, infinite dimensions, so if there are infinite dimensions why should countless types of sentient beings not exist as well? Beings with very high capacity and beings who are very weak. If we provoke them, those with higher capacities can send us a lot of negativity and this is what is called negative provocations. Sometimes they are directed at the family, who will pay to the end of the generation. We do not know how we provoke them because there are sentient beings that we can see and others that we cannot. If we walk in a garden we can see many small animals: some may see us, others do not. This is an example of the fact that there are beings with far more power than us, but that we cannot see: if we provoke them, of course they can send us some negativity. If we provoke a small animal, like a mouse, for example, it will at least try to bite us, it will provoke us in this way, while if it is larger, then the provocation will be much heavier.

So when there is a negative provocation in the illness, it is important to know how to control it. For example, for curing we also use mantras, words that contain a high potentiality and produce it through sound. After receiving transmission of them, by reciting them we can produce their function. This is one of the therapies, still in use today, of the ancient Bön tradition that was also using different kinds of rites. The ancient Bön tradition is very different from modern Bön.

For example, if a person has a disease linked to sentient beings such as the *nagas* (which indicates a negative provocation), instead of directly treating the person who is ill, they make contact with the *nagas* and in this way the person can overcome the illness. This is the way of seeing in the ancient Bön tradition, which also developed many rituals for healing, for having prosperity in the country and so on. Many people think that the Bön tradition is interesting because it has magical power, but today the greater part of the Bön has conformed to Buddhism, it only has the name "Bön" and does not have much knowledge of the ancient tradition or even accept it.

I understood this when I did my research. In my book *Drung Deu Bön* I explained twelve types of Bön. If you are interested in knowing the characteristics of the ancient Bön try to read it, it is already translated into Western languages. It is an interesting book. I wrote it because in Tibetan history, one wonders how the Tibetan kings had ruled Tibet for many generations before Songtsen Gampo without writing and it states that they did so through *drung deu bön*. But no one explains what they are so I thought it was important to do some research on the subject.

Drung is the narrative: there are various types of narrative, even if they are not written down. *Deu* is divination. These two aspects are not very difficult. What is more difficult, however, is the Bön. In Tibet at the time of the Tibetan kings all the Bön that existed in Shang Shung had not developed. The Bön that developed in Tibet was called *Bön Shepa Chunyi*, which means twelve knowledges of Bön. Each of these has its own characteristics: one concerns more astrology, another medicine, rituals, and so forth. One is called *cha bön,* which means to call the glory and increase it. Another is the *durshe sishen* and concerns rituals to be carried out when someone dies and for the preservation of the body, which was considered very important at the time of the Tibetan kings. One of them, the *shawa rugye* – *shawa* means deer – is somewhat complicated. Eventually I found two or three texts that explained something, but it was not entirely clear for me, whereas I explained very well the other Bön.

I also wrote another book called *The Light of Kailash (ti se 'i 'od zer),* in which I have divided the history of Tibet into three eras: the epoch of Shang Shung, the epoch of Shang Shung and Tibet, and the epoch of Tibet. This is *my* way of doing research.

The first is the epoch of Shang Shung. In that period the Tibetan kingdom did not exist, and the Tibetan people were divided in different tribes. But Shang Shung was very powerful at that time, it also dominated the Shang Shung Phugpa, today's Tagikistan and Kirgistan, countries that are now under Russia. In the history books of the Bön tradition they speak very much of Tazig. This is the actual Tagikistan, it is not Persia, as many people think, it has nothing to do with Persia. There was a very important teacher of Shang Shung, a Bönpo teacher called Trenpa Namkha. There were three Trenpa Namkhas. The first one was from Tazig, Tagikistan: he became student of Tönpa Shenrab and became a very important teacher of the Bön. After he passed away, since he had been an important teacher, another scholar from Shang Shung received the name Trenpa Namkha. This is the Trenpa Namkha of Shang Shung.

Also in the time of Guru Padmasambhava in Tibet, among his twenty-five students there was one called Lachen Trenpa Namkha who was originally Bön: this is the Trenpa Namkha of Tibet.

There is a collection of many books by Trenpa Namkha of Shang Shung, a kind of *terma* books of the Bön tradition: they consider these are originally from Trenpa Namkha. In any case they are very interesting books.

This is the background of Tibetan culture and history. Here we have excellent Tibetan doctors and in these days there are lectures. You should follow; this is very important occasion for you. For that reason I did not explain anything about the Tibetan medicine. We have a Tibetan saying: "When there is an ocean you do not use saliva to make a dry skin of an animal smooth."

Thank you very much for your attention.

PRESENTATION

KUNCHOK GYALTSEN
The Influence of Behavior and Lifestyle on Health

January 12, morning (10:30)

Good morning. Yesterday Dr. O, President of Arura Tibetan Medical Group, wanted to show you a PowerPoint presentation about Arura, but we could not arrange it. So, I will take a few minutes to show you what Arura is, and then I will move to my subject.

Arura is a Tibetan medical group based in Tibet, in the area traditionally known as Amdo. It is one of the biggest Tibetan medicine organizations in the world and has five major institutions. Doctor Outshon Tsokchen is the founder and president of the Arura Tibetan Medical Group.

Among the five institutions, the first is the University Tibetan Medical College, which is an educational training center. It is one of the major Tibetan medical colleges in China; currently, there are over 1,000 undergraduate students. The institution has formal Bachelor's and Master's degrees, as well as doctoral students. This is the only Tibetan medical institution that offers international degrees. Shang Shung Institute in America sends students to the medical school for their practicum and theoretical training; students are also sent to the Tibetan Medical Hospital.

The second institution is the Tibetan Medicine and Cultural Museums, which preserve, collect, and display over 20,000 items related to Tibetan medicine and culture. The displays include astrology, astronomy, Tibetan medicine *thangkas*, therapeutic objects, and ancient classical Tibetan medicine texts books. One of the displays is a 608 meter-long and 2.5 meter-wide *thangka* depicting Tibetan history from the original human development up until today's civilization. If you visit there, you need to set aside at least one day to see this *thangka*.

The third institution is the Provincial Tibetan Medical Hospital Inpatient Department. Currently it has 800 beds, with many patients from all over Tibet, as well as from China and overseas. The Tibetan Medicine Hospital provides both Tibetan and biomedical therapeutic modalities. One of the treatments is herbal baths, which is very effective for chronic issues like skin disease and arthritis.

The fourth organization is the Provincial Tibetan Medicine Research Institute. The function of this institute is primarily clinical research, laboratory research, and a project documenting related literature. As you know, prior to 1980, Tibetan medicine went through terribly difficult times. Now, in the past thirty years, we were able to adopt the study and practice of Tibetan medicine again. Currently, we have been able to publish over one hundred books on Tibetan medicine, which are classical Tibetan medicine texts. One of the projects we mentioned here yesterday is this collection of books, a 60-volume set called *Tibetan Medicine: An Extraordinary Collection of Classical Texts.* These textbooks were compiled from over 600 sources to form the highest quality collection on the subject of Tibetan medicine.

The content of this set includes a history of Tibetan medicine and commentaries in eight main components. In order to complete this set of books, more than a thousand Tibetan medical scholars from Amdo, Kham, and the western Tibetan regions were involved. As you know, before 1980 all the books were burned, destroyed, and the monasteries were destroyed. Tibetan Buddhist monks were put in jail, and many terrible things happened. In order to rebuild Tibetan medicine, we had to work very hard to find the resources from all over Tibet, and from all over the world.

Last night Chögyal Namkhai Norbu was saying that Tibetan culture and Tibetan history can be traced back more than 4,000 years. Tibetan medicine has a particularly long history tracing back to Shang Shung. Among traditional medicines, Tibetan medicine has the largest documented collection of classical books. In order to carry on Tibetan medicine, we have to work very hard to preserve the books, and there are still many books in western Tibet that need to be preserved. Tibetan medicine is not something as simple as folk medicine; it is a very sophisticated and complex field of medical scholarship. So if you are interested, try to study the Tibetan language and read those books.

The fifth institution is the Pharmaceutical Company, which is a modern standard pharmaceutical company that sells medicine throughout China. It currently produces 80 kinds of medicine, which are permitted by the Chinese food and drug administration and are sold on the Chinese market. This earns a lot of money to support Tibetan medical projects in Tibet. In the past thirty years we achieved remarkable success. Tibetan medicine is a universal treasure, and Dr. O, the President of Arura, very much admires and respects Chögyal Namkhai Norbu's overseas projects, so now we are working together and we want to establish more institutions overseas, like in America and Europe. One project we are working on is Arura Medicine of Tibet – established in Virginia, USA – to have training, medical treatment, research, wellness, and so on. In that way we can carry on the long-term development of Tibetan medicine in the future. This was a very brief introduction to Arura, and now I will move on to my subject.

Concept of Health

Tibetan medicine is a huge subject. We have only one hour (including translation), and it is impossible to cover everything. I will introduce the concept of health and how we can maintain health related with behavior.

The Tibetan medicine textbook *Gyüzhi*, the *Four Tantras*, says: "Oh, friend! Be sure to understand, those who wish to remain healthy and those who wish to cure others' illnesses must learn the healing system." This means that prevention is very important, more important than curing.

The first principle of Tibetan medicine is to remain healthy. If someone is not able to remain healthy, they will be ill and will need to be cured. That is the alternative. In a very brief concept: suppose after the birth there is no illness, Tibetan medicine would say we have a healthy body. So we have to remain healthy, we have to maintain our functions according to our life span and live longer. Each of us has a standard life span. When we reach that, we are considered to have lived long. If we have enough time in our life, then we can do a lot of good, positive things – which in Tibetan medicine we call Dharma – and can also succeed in creating wealth. As you see from Dharma, wealth actually is mental treasure and physical treasure. So, as human beings if we have both mental and physical wealth then we will be happy and reach human happiness. This is the perfect model of health. However, as human beings, every day we eat, drink, go around, sleep, do a lot of work, and we cannot maintain our health as we want. If in our body there is a little or a big problem – in Tibetan we call it *nyepa* – then we have to cure it or fix it. So, we see doctors in order to fix the problem and then we continue with our longevity on the normal track. Therefore, in Tibetan medicine, hospitals are less important than behavior, diet, and the daily life for health.

What makes our human body or mental body unhealthy or ill? There are four factors: time/location, obstacles, food/drink, and behavior. Those factors make a person's body become ill. We say the normal body becomes abnormal, which means *lung, tripa,* and *pekan* are altered. *Lung, tripa,* and *pekan* are the elements of the human body. We have to think about those four factors with which we are living in this complex environment. That is a challenge we face as human beings. Even though we have entitled today's lecture "Behavior and Lifestyle," we have to understand there is a more complex context. In order to achieve a healthy body and mind, we have to deal with this complex situation.

The Four Factors That Influence Our Health

So, the first one, which I mentioned earlier, is time. This is probably based on the Tibetan high altitude areas and seasonal differences and may be not applicable to Tenerife. Generally speaking, time differences very much affect our physical body. For example, summer versus winter, and spring versus fall: the four seasons. In Tibetan medicine we divide the year into six seasons, which very much applies to the Tibetan climate. Maybe I am wrong, but here in Tenerife you do not have seasonal changes, so you are very mellow. The reason time matters is that it affects our body very precisely, our body changes each season. To have a more precise description in terms of behavior and dietary changes, we divide the climate into six seasons.

And then, we have daytime; we have morning versus evening, midnight versus midday. Those timings affect the body very much; therefore, they are learned and studied in Tibetan astrology. As Chögyal Namkhai Norbu said last night, Tibetan medicine is very much related to astrology and astronomy. That is why in Tibetan we say *man* and *tsi*. *Man* is medicine and *tsi* is astrological calculations. Therefore, we have to understand cosmology, the earth, the moon, the sun, how the planets move around in different time, how that affects us. It is a huge body of knowledge.

Another aspect of time is environment, location: tropical area versus dry desert, forest versus grassland, and high versus low. Time has a strong effect on our health, so we must understand time well, and how the body changes with time.

The second factor is called *dön* in Tibetan. Sometimes it is translated in English as evil spirit. Here I call it obstacles, because it is more applicable in general. We can divide *dön* into different kinds. Some *dön* we can see with our human eyes, but some we cannot. For example, *dön* can be affected by anything. In Tibetan Buddhism scholars divide beings into six realms or dimensions: human beings, gods, demigods, hell beings, hungry ghosts, and animals. Some of you studied Buddhism and understand this well. What I am telling you is that in the cosmology in which we live, we are affected by each other. That is why as an individual, our health could be affected by anybody. Those are the obstacles.

For example, some people get sick when they meet a stranger. That is very similar to what they talk about as "evil eye" in South America. Human beings can affect each other in an abnormal way, which does not hurt physically, but energetically. Some of the beings move like human beings, move around in their circle, and then sometimes we hit them and we get sick. Usually those are car accidents, for example. There are spirits that move like this and then your car hits, because at that moment you see something very unusual, or sometimes you cannot control the way you want, that is why a lot of problems happen. I do not have precise statistics, but if you pay attention, those are the times when we have bad accidents. In our real life, we can see those experiences a lot. Some people are affected by spirits like hungry ghosts and go crazy. Some people can see things, see ghosts going around – we call them ghosts, but in the classification of ghosts there are a lot of ethnic groups, as among human beings. In Buddhist philosophy and cosmology, sentient beings are divided into three realms: the desire realm, the form realm, and the formless realm. In the latter, there is no physical body, but beings exist. Each type of being lives in their own world. For example, as human beings, the only other beings we see are animals. We do not see hungry ghosts, but we do see people who get sick, who desire to eat but cannot, similar to hungry ghosts. So, in the human dimension we see examples of all six dimensions, but the real dimensions also exist on different levels. Those different levels affect our physical body.

The third factor is diet, we call it *se. Se* includes food and drink. The day after tomorrow I will explain more. Today I will explain a little about the fourth one, behavior.

Physical Behavior

Usually we divide behavior into three: *gyunchöd* is the everyday behavior; it means you need to be careful all the time; *düchöpa* means you have to watch your behavior according to the season; and *nekab chölam* or circumstantial behavior means you have to behave according to circumstances. The general content is included in these three divisions, and this is how they are classified in Tibetan medical textbooks.

According to the first point, it is necessary to be taking care of the body according to seasonal conditions, in terms of low altitude and high altitude. For example, we never think about wearing clothes: you have to put on more clothes when you get cold; when you are hot, you put on fewer clothes. This is actually a part of healthy behavior, but we never think of it as medically relevant. There are a lot of details, but I am just picking some examples that may be useful for you. Regarding clothes, fabrics like nylon or other synthetic materials are not good for the body. You must be careful not to wear rubber-soled shoes too much. Particularly for young women – I see that here the audience is predominantly female – if you wear rubber-soled shoes, when you get pregnant and also during the menopause you will get a lot of symptoms, like lower back pain, and a lot of gas. These kinds of symptoms will show up. Usually if you wear leather-soled shoes, this is very good. And cotton is very good. Wearing them under the sun – in a very dry climate –is very healthy.

As regards our physical body: some people are skinny, some people are a little bit fat. So what do you do? The skinny ones need oil massage; it is very good for them. When they get oil massage, they can relax and sleep well. Fat people – I cannot say fat in America, but maybe here it is okay – need more exercise, and skinny people less exercise. In the West, at least in America, they use the wrong concept because exercise is not good all the time: only people who are heavy need exercise. People who are skinny should not do very much exercise. Fat people need dry massage; it is good for them, so in Tibet we use *tsampa*, barley flour.

Then, it is important to protect your eyes. Never wash your head or hair with hot water; you need to use cooler water. Those are some examples of how to behave, but there are a lot of details. In the future you can invite Doctor Phuntsog to have serious courses and then you will learn. I am sorry that I cannot cover everything in such a short time. In Tibet, Tibetan medicine is for scholars, it is not for the public. To understand these topics you have to put in a lot of effort, then you can learn. It is also not easy for us to make you understand with simple explanations.

Mental Behavior

Then, the second part of behavior, which is mental behavior, is more important than the physical. Later on you will hear from Dr. Lhusham Gyal about mental health, but now I want to emphasize two things we have to consider: *michöd,* humanity, and *lhachöd,* which means the behavior of heavenly beings. This humanity is actually right communication with other people. You have to speak properly, you have to behave properly, you need to be careful with bad people, and know how to treat good people. All those things are included here. In Tibetan we say that *michöd* is anything you achieve, that is the foundation. Therefore, you need to be a good person. Being a good person creates a lot of good opportunities for you, makes you happy and confident, and this becomes the foundation of your success in health.

Lhachöd is a more noble learning and noble behavior, which is actually very much related to Buddhist philosophy. Here in the Dzogchen Community a lot of people study Buddhist philosophy with Chögyal Namkhai Norbu and also do practice, so every day they remind themselves about *lhachöd.* So, those are exactly the things recommended in Tibetan medicine.

There are three levels in doing this. First you meet a good teacher. A good, qualified teacher is very important. You respect this teacher, you study with him or her, and you gain knowledge. When you gain knowledge, you are empowered in wisdom. Then what you do corresponds with what you practice. When you practice it means that if you are a bad person, you become a good person; if you are a good person, you become a better person; if you are a better person, you become the best person. This means that mentally and physically you need to be capable. That is the achievement of the second level.

Then the third level is based on the second level. You have those practices and then your mind becomes wider, which is the practice of compassion. Compassion in Tibetan Buddhism is not looking at yourself. You look at every sentient being, and say: "All sentient beings desire to have happiness, they do not want anything negative. Everybody wants to have happiness. What can I do? Maybe not everybody is achieving happiness. So I will accelerate my development as an instrument to lead them to achieve happiness." You have to have this kind of mental compassion.

Some Western scholars say that Buddhism is not a religion, but more like a philosophy, which is true. When you study and practice Dzogchen, for example, it sounds like you are following a religion, but in Buddhist philosophy we believe that it does not belong to anybody in particular; rather, it belongs to everybody. Just like food: anyone can come to enjoy food. When you have this knowledge, this wisdom, and then empower yourself, you can be of more benefit and very useful for human society. When you achieve that level, mentally you are very capable. Then, when you have a cancer or you have a terrible situation or experience, you understand better than anybody else. So, mentally we have to make ourselves strong. Therefore, every day we should be careful with our food and behavior, and then we will be very healthy. Considering all these factors, doctors could not fix the problem. Nurses could not fix problem. It is the same anywhere. We ourselves can learn and can fix our own situation. When we study more we have to learn the ten virtues. For example, how you behave in your speech. How you behave with your physical body. How you behave in your thinking. So, you include these three behaviors. The reason is that our physical body interacts with our mind and our mind, through the physical body, interacts with the five senses. The five senses go through speech, body and thinking, all of us have these three. Therefore we can communicate with each other. In this bigger environment we have to understand this, then we know where we are, so then we can practice our healthy way of being and that maintains our health of body and health of mind.

This is just a brief introduction I wanted to share with you. Now we have a few minutes, so you can ask questions.

Q: You were talking about the body we arrived with when we are born – a healthy body at birth. What about people who do not arrive with a healthy body?

A: You asked a very good question. Last night Chögyal Namkhai Norbu was saying: "What comes first, the chicken or the egg?" When I was talking it was theory. Theory is based on assumptions: we suppose that everybody started healthy. Of course, our life is not just this one. Particularly in Buddhist philosophy we had infinite lives before. Therefore, we collected karma, in Tibetan *le*. Every day we act with our physical body and collect karma. Every day we speak and collect karma. Every day we think and collect karma. It can be negative and positive. Basically negative things bring bad things to our life, ill health, sickness, and all those things. Positive things bring happiness, good health. Because of their karma many people are disabled. They cannot maintain their own health. Therefore, healthy and smart people study and then act. Then we influence other people to be healthy. That is also one of the aspects of compassion. That we emphasize.

Q: Can you say a little more about rubber-soled shoes?

A: Unfortunately, almost all shoes have rubber in the soles these days. Rubber creates heat. The heat does not go through the sole, it gets stuck there. Our feet in particular actually need to be warm, without the humidity of rubber. Therefore, any kind of rubber under the shoes is not good for our health at all. Especially if you wear rain boots, then you will feel that you have lower back pain. Unfortunately, shoes with leather or cotton soles are very difficult to find. But it is something we need to understand. Tibetan medicine understands this, so we need to speak out. Companies should not make rubber shoes. We can ask them to make healthy shoes, so we can wear healthy shoes and be healthier. If there are any scientists or researchers among you, you can test this hypothesis.

Q: How appropriate is Tibetan medicine for non-Tibetan cultures?

A: This is a very good question, a lot of people ask this question. Tibetan medicine was developed for the Tibetan population on the Tibetan plateau. It has a lot of rich information that other cultures can adapt. In order to adapt, *you* are the people who must study. Like us, we are just ambassadors, we are not real teachers here, because we just give a brief introduction. Western people need to study, and then adapt it to their language, to their cultures. And then, in the future, it will become part of your culture and will be of more benefit. Why do I say this? Because we have examples like Tibetan Buddhism. Buddhism came from India. Even though they are from the same region, Indian culture and Tibetan culture are very different. But Tibetans lived in India, studied Sanskrit and translated texts into Tibetan and then also practiced in the Tibetan context. Then, many became great teachers. They started to write book after book, and now Tibetan Buddhism is the most complex field of Buddhist studies in the world. Similarly, if you want to have Tibetan medicine here in the West, you have to study and make it your own, and then it will become real. Otherwise, the Tibetan way is not appropriate here, and there can be a lot of intercultural problems. Actually, Tibetan medicine has a very complex theory and deep understanding of human beings, not only from Tibetan areas. It is universal. Therefore, it is very easy to apply to in any kind of society and region. That is why Tibetan culture, and particularly medicine and Buddhist philosophy, are very valuable treasures for human beings. That is why we need to carry on, we cannot lose it. In Chögyal Namkhai Norbu's words last night: "Tibetan culture is important for everybody, not only for Tibetans." A lot of Tibetan medicine techniques can be used easily in the West. But if you are talking on a bigger scale, we would like you to study Tibetan language and study real Tibetan medicine. And then translate into Spanish and practice here. Then, it will be part of your culture, your medical system, and will help people here.

Thank you very much. Doctor Lhusham Gyal will present the next lecture.

PRESENTATION

LHUSHAM GYAL
Dealing with Mental Illnesses from the Perspective of Tibetan Medicine

January 12, morning (11:30)

First of all I would like to thank everybody attending the Tibetan Event Week and the four Arura members and particularly I would like to thank all the audience present today to listen to our talk because this for me is an opportunity to be together and to discuss Tibetan medicine.

Today my topic is Tibetan psychology, how to perform a clinical diagnosis, and how to treat. I am going to discuss three topics: what is consciousness in Tibetan medicine or in Buddhism; what is mind and where is the mental function located; and what is its support or base.

The second topic is how to distinguish the healthy or balanced mind from the unhealthy or unbalanced mind, and what the factors and concepts involved in this lack of balance are.

The third topic is the clinical aspect: disease, its causes, its conditions, its symptoms, and how to treat it.

In general, within the framework of Tibetan Buddhism, we summarize the various aspects of phenomena in three categories, the direct, the indirect, and the inner indirect, also called the outer, inner, and secret aspects. The same terms are used when we discuss the concept of consciousness.

The first or outer aspect is when we use our five sense organs to perceive, for example to hear, see, or smell. Anything can appear to our sense organs; this is called direct contact or the outer aspect.

The second or inner aspect, also called indirect, is when the five sense organs cannot see, hear, or smell something directly because although it exists it is beyond the range the senses are able to perceive.

The third aspect we call secret or inner indirect. This means contact between your sense organs and the object is impossible; you cannot perceive it or even imagine it. This we call the deeper or secret aspect. This can only be perceived by extraordinary and special beings but not by ordinary people.

In Tibetan medicine and Buddhism, in explanations pertaining to the mind we call the three aspects of its functioning direct, indirect, and inner indirect.

The mental function or consciousness is often said to be located or have its base in the brain or in the sense organs. Since with these we can perceive or have contact of the senses with objects, we categorize them as the outer aspect. But when we refer to things that are more connected with the heart or the chakras, these pertain to the inner or indirect aspect, since we can think about them or try to feel them but obviously they are not something we can contact directly.

On a still deeper level than the chakras are the three principal channels: *uma*, *kyangma*, and *roma*. We refer to this aspect as inner indirect.

What we have discussed before is the origin or source of the mind, where it is based. Talking in general about what the mind is, we say it brings us the feeling of happiness or unhappiness, of good and bad. These kinds of feelings spring from the mind, as this is its action or its nature.

So this is the mind, this is consciousness. The mind not perturbed by secondary causes is pure and transparent, like water. It is said it has the nature of emptiness. If the mind is conditioned by the presence of some secondary conditions or causes like hatred, attachment, or ignorance, and so on, that leads to impurity, which means it is like water polluted and murky, not pure and transparent. The first slide shows the consciousness is located or based in the brain and in the sense organs and this information is similar to that explained by modern science. In the brain there is a channel called *kyilwa* and consciousness is based in this channel and in the function of the sense organs. Thus in general, there is *kyilwa* which means life-sustaining channel, with 500 channels based on it, connected to the function of the sense organs. It has three functions or aspects, the first is conditioned, the second is unconditioned, and the third is more specific, the secret part.

If we explain these three concepts a little more in depth, the first one is the *dakyen*. If we take, for example, the eyes or vision, vision refers to the concept of seeing outer objects. The second one is *migkyen*, which refers to a field of perception in which there is a form or color. Then *demadakyen* is the secret part. Thus with a field of perception plus your own sense organs, the two – object and subject – mix together, producing in you a feeling born from information going to the brain. Once you have these three functions, the sense organs or subject, the field of perception or object, and the third condition, the coming together of the first two, and once you practice and train your mind little by little directing it ever more toward positive actions, then eventually you can reach enlightenment.

The second aspect we described earlier is the consciousness that is like a heartbeat in the heart chakra. The channel called *yesangma* is located in the physical heart, and through it moves the wind element, corresponding to the circulation of the blood. This is symbolized by the 500 channels that spring from the heart and through which emotions function.

The third one is the consciousness based on the chakras. In Tibetan medicine where do we think the consciousness is based? It is based in the wind. Where is the wind element based? It is based in the channels.

Where are the channels based? The channels are based in the body. That is why it is very important to study yoga or *thrulkor*, like Yantra Yoga, and anatomy and the bodily functions.

What you see in this slide are the five chakras. The first chakra is called the chakra of happiness; it is in the crown chakra and is based on thirty-two channels. The second one is the throat chakra that we call the enjoyment chakra and is based on sixteen channels. The third one is the heart chakra, called dharma chakra, and is based on eight channels. The fourth chakra is called the navel chakra and is based on sixty-four channels. The last is the secret chakra and is based on thirty-two channels. Thus there are five chakras and three principal channels, which are the central channel and the left and right ones, which are *kyangma* and *roma*. These are just concepts; it does not mean that the five chakras correspond to something on a physical plane. These chakras can be felt when you practice yoga but cannot be seen at an anatomical level.

So far we have discussed the three aspects of the mental function. The first one is that the consciousness is based on the brain and the sense organs. The second is that the consciousness is based or located in the heart chakra and all the emotional gates. The third is that the consciousness flows through the chakras and the three major channels, the central, left, and right. Thus basically all the mental concepts are covered.

Healthy or Unhealthy Mind

At this moment to summarize and make it easier to understand, we leave the chakra system as it is explained in the yoga system and we focus on the brain aspect and then on the heart in its aspect of an emotional gate.

Consciousness includes six major or main aspects of the mind, which are the five sense organs plus the central consciousness. Then there are fifty-one secondary mental concepts so that we have two aspects: the major mental concepts and the secondary mental concepts.

Studying consciousness, we learn first that its base or subtle consciousness is called *kunzhi nampar shepa*. Second is again the emotional aspect. The third one is more like the memory, the mental aspect. The fourth one is the concept of the sense organs. All this starts from the subtle and goes toward the more material and when we get to the sense organs all is very concrete.

When we speak of mental consciousness, we talk of the six or eight emotions. If the eight are summarized into six it is fine, because they are derived from the five sense organs and the central consciousness. Based on the six major or main consciousnesses or concepts, there are fifty-one secondary ones. What are they? The first five are preliminary, the next [26] are major, and the last twenty are secondary, in this way totaling fifty-one. In the relationship between the body and the mind, the mind is like the owner and the body is like the assistant. The difference is that the main mental concepts act like a king and the secondary mental concepts act like ministers. When we talk about disease in Tibetan medicine, all diseases are affected or involved with the mental aspects. The mental does not refer to the secondary fifty-one mental aspects, but to the six main ones. In these six mental concepts, one of the main ones is called the *yighe nampar shepa* or *yighe yeshe*. Not only the psychological diseases are based on the mental, but also the physical diseases are involved or affected by the mental. How? For example, if you see something beautiful or attractive, or you hear something nice or smell something pleasant or taste something delicious, anything that makes you happy leads to happiness and happiness leads to health. And on the contrary, that which you dislike or see as ugly or bad can lead to unhappiness. One we call positive, the other negative. If something neither leads you to happiness nor to unhappiness it is called neutral. Therefore, your outer concepts lead you to happiness, to unhappiness, or are neutral; based on that we have the so-called three poisons in Tibetan Buddhism, which are hatred, attachment, and ignorance. These three poisons result in the three *nyepa*, which means the three faults. All the diseases are based on these three faults, i.e. *lung* (wind), *tripa* (bile), and *pekan* (phlegm).

As we said before, we can divide the mental negative concepts into three poisons: hatred, attachment, and ignorance. These, in turn, can be summarized as *marigpa* or ignorance, through which we can accumulate 84,000 negative concepts. How can we find an antidote to these negative concepts or how can we heal those sufferings? If you look at the outer or material level the antidote to those 84,000 mental sufferings, or more simply the three poisons, is not easy to locate. You also need to find the antidote to your mind through your mind. The Buddha taught 84,000 volumes of teachings with the purpose of applying antidotes to those 84,000 negative mental actions.

As we said before, all causes of suffering are created by the three poisons hatred, attachment, and ignorance. Through these three aspects the 84,000 sufferings or emotions are created. Through these all the diseases appear. Sakya Pandita, the great scholar of the Sakya tradition, said: "If you have enemies and want to control all of them you cannot. But if you try to control or conquer your own enemy, that is, ignorance or hatred, it is equivalent to subjugating all your enemies." That means that if you try to kill the enemies outside, there is no end to enemies; trying instead to conquer your enemies inside has much more value and effect.

Tibetan medicine considers that each disease has its own condition or cause but its primary or original cause is the three poisons. Attachment, hatred, and ignorance lead to all suffering and diseases. In particular, attachment leads to *lung* disorder, hatred leads to *tripa* disorder, and ignorance leads to *pekan* disorder. We are not only just saying this: it is backed by proof arrived at through research. For example, when we say that attachment leads to wind or produces the wind element or the *lung* disorder, this is based on the location of the disorder creating winds in the body, and how the wind channel is formed, and thirdly what its action is. That attachment produces the wind disorders is confirmed by a strong base of research corroborated by much observation.

The Clinical Disease

What we explained until now is the mental aspect in the understanding of Tibetan medicine. Now I am going to explain the clinical disease that we call *soglung* in Tibetan. The primary symptom of *soglung* is anxiety: the person becomes very unstable, which means he or she continuously moves a lot, coming and going, and also sighs frequently, takes long breaths, talks a lot of nonsense, and is also unable to sleep. That means that body, mind, and speech all become unstable. Why do we have these types of symptoms? Especially today in modern society and in the so-called developed countries everything is growing very fast; everything has become very stressful and there is much competition between person and person or society and society or community and community. That brings the individual heavy stress, which causes all these problems. Therefore, again the cause is ignorance.

To make things clear, there are four conditions: diet, behavior, season, and provocations or obstacles. Behaviors that can lead to mental disease are for example if you work too much, talk too much, undergo heavy suffering or mourning, or your mind is too focused on something.

What kind of food makes you anxious or leads to unhappiness? Eating or drinking much food with a bitter taste – coffee or tea – can also lead to an excess of the wind element. Again, talking about the nature of food, which kinds can increase mental problems? For example, too much raw or light food can do so. This does not mean that if you have a cup of coffee today, tomorrow you will have mental symptoms. But if you use a certain taste or type of food in excess – either using it for a long time or one time in a big quantity – that excess amount can create a problem.

When we refer to conditions based on the time of year, we mean an excess or a deficiency or a disturbance of the season: for example, if the summer is much hotter or cooler than usual the imbalance between temperature and season can also cause disease. Among the four seasons, the season that most aggravates these mental symptoms is summer or the rainy season; and in the span of the day it is the late afternoon and early morning.

Another condition that causes disease is the *dön*, which Dr. Gyaltsen explained earlier as obstacles or provocations. Here also we can have different obstacles or negative things for *lung* disorder, but one of them is if you have a sudden shock or fear, that also can cause a *lung* disorder, such as mental anxiety.

Summarizing, these types of diseases, called *soglung* in Tibetan medicine, are a malfunction of the life-sustaining wind. The life-sustaining channel is located in the brain: this means that the brain function is affected. In our modern society, not so many people are seriously sick with *soglung*. If one is seriously sick, it means one is crazy and ends up in a mental institution. The seriously ill are not that many, but a lot of people are affected in a minor way, especially people in offices who do no physical work, but rather overwork their brain where the *soglung* is located.

If we check where these kinds of problems are more diffused, in the East or in the West, we see they are more common in the West. In the East, they are more present in China and Japan: this means life in these countries is more stressful. In China and Western countries we can see more of these kinds of problems because there is a lot of competition and stress in life there. In Tibet there is less: one reason could be because there is less stress, and another can be that we are helped by our religion and Buddhist culture which makes us calmer.

Treatment

How can we treat these types of diseases or how can we prevent them if we do not want to become sick? Again with four things: diet, behavior, medicine, and external therapies. Diet concerns eating food and drinking liquids. When considering the nature of food, which is good for these kinds of diseases, any kind of heavy, oily, and smooth foods, that is, those with a sweet or salty taste are good. Dairy products, like milk, yogurt, cheese, and butter also basically have a sweet taste and are good. So all dairy products, and sweet products like molasses, honey, sugar, and that type of food are also good. If you have these sorts of problems, warm-natured food is also good such as spices like cardamom, nutmeg, black pepper, or long pepper. If someone has difficulty to sleep, one-and-a-half or two hours before going to sleep warm up some milk with cardamom or long or black pepper and drink it and then go to sleep. That helps one be able to sleep.

As for the medicines, medicines with agar, myrobalan, and also those based on nutmeg and on cardamom are good. In Tibetan medicine we have many medicines with agar, like agar 20, 15, 30, and 31, and many formulas contain myrobalan as well.

As for external therapies, oil treatment is good. You can do some Kunye oil massage or you can have warm oil compresses and also warm oil massage. If you receive a warm oil compress or moxibustion treatment, you need to do it on the *lung* points. If you have a professional do it for you it is great; otherwise you can also do it yourself, massaging certain points.

As regards behavior, it is also based on body, mind, and speech. Today I would like to focus on the mind, so meditation is very good and very effective. I know here there are many Community member students of Chögyal Namkhai Norbu, so I am sure you are doing much practice and meditation. Meditation is very good.

When we talk of meditation, I am sure that the Dzogchen Community people have received teachings and instructions from Chögyal Namkhai Norbu. Generally there are many methods of meditation but the most common is Shine, which is fixation meditation. If you have this kind of problem it is good to do Shine meditation, best if you can do it four times a day or, if you do not have time, three, or two times, like in the morning and evening. If you do not have time, at least do it once a day before going to sleep. When you do it, try to first eliminate all impure breath and try to inhale fresh air and then try to calm down your mind. When we do meditation, it is very important to receive the empowerment transmission from your teacher. I am sure Chögyal

Namkhai Norbu taught these things: it is very important when you do meditation that you manifest living compassion. Compassion is the most important factor when you meditate because through it you accumulate good merits.

Thank you very much for listening.

Q: Could you explain the role of *marigpa* or ignorance in mental illness?

A: *Marigpa* can be explained in many ways. As I said before, our mind when it is not enmeshed in emotions or conflicts is pure and transparent like water, but in many lifetimes it has been affected by bad karmic acts and has become polluted. Even if mind is pure and transparent and has the seed of Buddha nature, we cannot see its purity and luminosity. That is because of ignorance. Without seeing or knowing, your ignorance leads you to continue samsaric negative actions, and you continue to be in samsara. At a simple level, if you do not pay attention and follow daily life necessities properly – like rules of social conduct or daily diet – ignorance can lead you to end up in jail or in the hospital. This is also part of ignorance. Ignorance can be explained on many levels. *Rig* means seeing, *marig* means not seeing. What you are not seeing is yourself: it means not seeing what you do, therefore not seeing your condition.

PRESENTATION

PHUNTSOG WANGMO *and* FABIO ANDRICO
The Practice of Yantra Yoga for a Correct Balance Between Mind, Energy, and Body

January 12, afternoon

Phuntsog Wangmo

First of all I would like to say I am very happy to be here with you today. Also I would like to thank all the Shang Shung team, the organizers, sponsors, collaborators and, in particular, our dear Master Chögyal Namkhai Norbu, who's tireless work has brought us together here to discuss Tibetan culture. As Chögyal Namkhai Norbu said yesterday, Tibetan medicine and culture are of benefit not only for Tibetans but also for all sentient beings and communities.

Some of you may know about Tibetan culture while for others it is something new. Tibetan medicine is similar to conventional medicine. When we talk about medicine there are two aims: prevention and treatment. In Tibetan medicine the way of prevention and treatment is through the theory of the five elements. As I said, the aim of all types of medicine is the same but the approach is slightly different. Tibetan medicine is based on the theory of the five elements, meaning that all phenomena are composed of the five elements, the outer and inner elements: earth, water, fire, wind or air, and space. The first four elements are the material substances that form the body. The last one, space, is not material, but empty and gives the opportunity to the other elements to develop. This is the origin of our material body. What is the correspondence of the five elements to our body? We will discuss this tomorrow morning in the section on conception and embryology.

Today we will try to focus more on the cause of disease and how we treat it. In Tibetan medicine we have already said that the function of the five elements is the development of our body, but what do we need in order to regenerate or maintain it? Again, we need the five elemental substances.

The Five Elements

One of the elements is wind, which refers to all of our movements, including inhaling, exhaling, etc. Once we have inhaled, what is the purpose of the inhalation and the benefit for our body, which is made up of the earth element? Wind benefits the movement of the earth element. Once the earth element moves, we need the fire element to regenerate or mature it. The three elements of fire, wind, and earth together are dry and something cohesive is needed. To smoothen we need the water element. For example, if we plant a flower firstly we need a seed, but in order to grow, the seed needs some soil. Soil is the earth element. When we have the seed and soil, do we have a flower? No, we also need water, because otherwise the soil will not mature the seed. So we need the water element. Once soil and water are together it becomes mud, which is heavy and cold and does not produce anything. Then we need the fire element to produce heat in order to make it grow. Perhaps in this part of the world you do not have much experience because the four seasons here are quite stable. But in other countries like in my country, Tibet, farmers do not cultivate crops in the wintertime because there is not enough heat.

Once we have these three elements – earth, water, and fire – this is still not enough to grow a flower: we need the air element to move, to stimulate growth. And the last element we require in order for a flower to grow is space; otherwise nothing will grow.

As for the outer nature, our body also needs to grow: so all five elements are important. When the five elements are healthy and balanced, we have a healthy body and a happy mind; when they are unbalanced, we are unhealthy and unhappy. In Tibetan we call medicine *man*, which means benefit. *Man* does not refer to pills or herbs, techniques or treatments, it is something that benefits the body by keeping it healthy and happy.

When we consider Dharma (Buddhism), or yoga, or when we eat and drink, when we undertake any movement, everything is part of medicine, part of health. In everything we do or plan or endeavor, we try to be healthy and happy. Nevertheless, if certain movements we do are wrong, we will have unexpected results.

We eat in order to have good health and regenerate our body. If we observe, either we do some positive action or negative action, but whatever we do we are trying to attain health and happiness. However sometimes we do wrong actions or have a wrong diet and that makes us unhappy and we have unexpected results. So, the understanding of our body and the study of yoga are interdependent. If you want to study medicine without understanding yoga or if you want to study yoga without understanding medicine it will not work out well. Some people do yoga and the result is that they cannot sleep or cannot move the body. These people might think that something bad has happened from doing yoga, but that has nothing to do with yoga. The problem is that they did not understand their body.

Similarly someone might think that eating certain food has made him or her ill. The problem is not with the food but that they do not understand their body. So, since our body is made up of the five elements, in order to keep them balanced we need to know how to work with them.

When we consider our breathing, for example, if we breathe too much we do not feel better, but if we do not breathe we know what the result will be. The same with food: in general it is regenerative, but if we eat too much it does not make us happy. So, it is important that everything is balanced.

When we talk about balance it is important that the five elements are balanced, but most of all the wind element because the nature of the wind element is very light, very rough, and very subtle. It is also very unstable. This means that if you have an excess of wind this can lead to disease. Wind can also make a disease spread more quickly since it moves more quickly than other elements, especially earth and water. On the other hand, all our movements are based on wind: inhaling and exhaling, having thoughts, opening and closing our sense organs are all related to wind. Most of the actions of the body depend on wind. And where does wind go? As we said before wind is subtle, so it goes everywhere and for this reason when we do yoga an important part of it is the breathing. Our main Yantra Yoga instructor Fabio Andrico is going to talk about that. What I am explaining today is more the physical aspects.

The Five Types of Wind Element

There is one general wind element under five subcategories. The first, the life-sustaining wind, is located in the crown chakra, more specifically in the central nerve, which is called the life-sustaining channel. It travels down through the throat to the chest and its action or function is to give us the ability to swallow and inhale and to produce saliva and sneezing.

The second wind is the ascending wind. It is located in the chest and goes up through the chest and throat to the nose. The main functions of this wind are to form words when we speak, clarify our memory, give strength to our body (not only physical strength but more inner strength), and promote determination.

The third wind is located in the heart and moves with the blood circulation throughout the whole body. Its function is to move the whole body, so it is related to all movements like stretching, opening, and closing.

The fourth wind is located in the stomach. We say stomach, but it is more in the large intestine because it goes from the stomach to the rectum, including all the digestive tract, approximately a length of 2.5 meters, and back to the stomach and all the digestive area. When we ingest food this wind helps to digest it by making the heat a little stronger so we can digest more quickly. In addition to digestion, it also aids the process of extracting the food and dividing it into pure and impure.

The last is the descending wind, which is located in the pelvic area and goes into the reproductive organs, bladder, and inner thighs. The functions of this wind are to open or close, for example, opening for urination and then closing. These functions also include the actions related to sperm, egg, menstruation, and labor.

These are the five subcategories of the wind element.

The Five Types of the Earth and Water Elements

What do the earth and water elements do? We put these elements together because they are both heavy, dull, and have a cold nature. There are also five subcategories.

The first we call *pekan tengye*, the supporting phlegm, which is located in the chest and whose function is to produce all the liquids and lubrication in our body and also support the water and earth elements.

The second one is called *pekan nyagye*, the decomposing phlegm, and is located in the upper part of the stomach, near the esophagus. Its function is to make the food smooth when it reaches the stomach and grind it to make it sticky.

The third is the *pekan tsimgye,* the satisfying *pekan.* It is located in the brain and satisfies the actions of the other *pekan* especially the sense organs. So when we eat, see, speak, whatever we do or whatever contact we have with the outer nature, it gives us a boundary that tells us: "That is enough."

The fourth one we call *pekan nyongye,* the tasting phlegm. It is located in the tongue and its function is to distinguish taste. Taste is very important whether we talk of balancing the body or treating it. We can say that a taste is good or not.

As regards taste there are six tastes: sweet, sour, salty, bitter, hot, and astringent. Why do we need to know tastes? Each taste is composed of two elements. This does not mean that other elements are not present, but that two elements are predominant.

The sweet taste is predominated by the earth and water elements. Sour taste is predominated by the earth and fire elements. Salty taste is predominated by the water and fire elements. Bitter taste is predominated by the wind and water elements. Hot taste is predominated by the fire and wind elements. Astringent taste is predominated by the earth and wind elements. Therefore, two elements combine to make one taste: the *pekan nyongye*, or tasting phlegm, is located in the tongue and distinguishes these tastes.

The last *pekan* is the *pekan jyorgye*, or connecting phlegm. It is located in the joints and its function is to move the joints and connect the upper and lower part of the body and the parts of the joints.

These are the five inner aspects or inner functions or subcategories of the earth and water elements.

The Five Types of the Fire Element

As regards the fire element there are also five subcategories. The first one is the *tripa jugye*, or digestive bile, which is located in the stomach near the duodenum. Its function is to digest after the decomposing phlegm has decomposed food, descending down to the bile then helping to mature and extract the essence.

The second *tripa* is the *tripa drubgye*, which means accomplishing bile. It is located in the heart *chakra* and its function is to give inner strength, determination, a sharp mind, and overall intelligence.

The third is the *tripa dangyur*, changing-color bile, located in the liver. When it receives the essence of the food, its function is to change its colors into the next step. Our bodies function through the seven substances. Six of them – blood, muscles, fat, bones, bone marrow, and reproductive fluids – come from the essence of food or chyle. Together they make up the seven constituents, which make our body function. Each step changes the color of each substance, which is why it is called the changing-color bile.

The fourth is *tripa thongye*, the sight-giving bile. It is located in the eyes and helps us to distinguish forms, colors, and have all the functions of vision.

The fifth bile is *tripa dogsal*, the clearing-color bile. It is located in the skin and its function is to keep our skin clear. It also functions automatically: in wintertime it closes the pores to keep the heat inside the body, while in summer it opens the pores to exchange air with the outside.

These are the five biles of the fire element.

We use these four terms – wind, earth, water, and fire elements – when we talk about how to conceive or build the body. However, when we talk about disease or pathology, we use the terms *lung, tripa*, and *pekan*: *lung* is the wind element, *tripa* is the fire element, *pekan* is a combination of the earth and water elements. We speak about *lung* and *tripa* first of all because wind and fire are sharp and fast and clinically more critical. *Pekan* comes last.

The Purpose of Yoga

At this point you can understand why we do yoga and what its purpose is. Since our body is composed of the five elements, maintained by the five elements, and works with the five elements, if we wish to maintain the five body elements, we need to eat and drink. Everybody knows that.

But people do not pay attention to the breath, which is even more critical than eating and drinking. We can survive a few days without food or water, but it is impossible to remain even two or three minutes without breathing. Not many people consider that breathing is part of life, that it is very important for maintaining the body. When we are sick everybody knows we should see a doctor and get some medicine, but not many people pay attention to or think that if they try to change their breathing a little or to coordinate it that is part of health just like medicine and treatment.

We have a saying in Tibet: "If you live too close to something you cannot see it or you do not think it is important." Our eyebrows are very close to our eyes, but normally we do not see them. It is the same with breathing. It is a very important part of life, but people do not pay attention to it. It is a very important aspect of treatment, but people do not realize it.

On the other hand, some people think that yoga is very important, that breathing is very important, and that they should do it as much as they can. Yet they do not consider that our body is also made up of other elements, such as earth, water, and fire. So if breathing is important, exercise is too, and in the meantime we should not forget the earth and water elements. As I said, the nature of wind is light: if we have too much wind it means too much lightness. Wind is part of creating thoughts, the action of wind makes you think, yet if you have too many thoughts that is also not necessarily good.

The earth and water elements are like a base, a heavy substance, and beneficial to remaining calm and stable. However, being overly calm is also not necessarily good.

Fire is determination, sharpness, and gives self-confidence, yet too much sharpness or intelligence is not necessarily good. It is important that everything is balanced.

Balance can be reached through diet and also through breathing and movement. This is what we call behavior.

Now I will pass you on to Fabio Andrico, who will explain about movements and breathing.

Fabio Andrico

I also want to start by thanking our Teacher, Chögyal Namkhai Norbu, who has very generously opened the doors of his boundless knowledge to us, and I would like to thank everybody who participated in making this event possible and is still working for that.

As Doctor Phuntsog said and focused on, the aspect of breathing is essential for the practice of Yantra Yoga. Somehow Yantra Yoga is designed around different aspects of the breathing. We should understand that there is not only the quantity of the breathing but there is also the *quality* of the breathing. There is not only the more material aspect of the function of the breathing, but there is the aspect of the function of the breathing related to the condition of our energy.

Very often the different systems of yoga that we see in the Western world are very much focused on anatomy, on the alignment of positions. All this is good, all the aspects related with the physical body are good. But, from what I have understood from Tibetan medicine, the understanding of anatomy is not limited only to the physical aspects of bones, muscles, and so on. There is a kind of anatomy of the energy, an understanding of how the energy travels through our condition. As a matter of fact, the condition of the energy is an extremely important and fundamental part of the practice of Yantra Yoga.

Energy moves. Our life moves. So, it is very important that we know how to deal with this movement, that we know how to coordinate and harmonize this aspect. That basically is what the practice of Yantra Yoga is. The practice of Yantra Yoga is integrating the movement in the aspect of our condition, our breathing and the condition of our mind, coordinating, balancing, and harmonizing the function of the elements.

As I said before, beyond the quantity of the breathing, we also have to consider the *quality*. There are different functions of the wind and people also have some understanding. For example, the most well known word is *prana* and today everybody knows what *prana* is. There is even a company called Prana that makes yoga clothing. So, somehow there is an understanding of something that is also external. My Hatha Yoga teacher in India used to say that it is better to go to a high mountain with nice pine trees, because there you can feel that the air is full of *prana*. Then the techniques of breathing in yoga are very often called *pranayama*. The interpretation of my teacher was to take the *prana* in. But, as Doctor Phuntsog explained, and also from the point of view of Tibetan medicine, there is an internal function of the *prana* and there are ways in which different kinds of aspects of the channels work with functions of the *prana* and *prana* traveling and there is a whole anatomy that is different from the one that we can *see* with material instruments that is not easy to understand without another point of view.

Nowadays we are more familiar with therapies like acupuncture, which works with the principles of channels – vehicles of energy that moves – that are blocked or need to be released or that are too concentrated or weak. But what happens is that, not only from the point of view of Tibetan medicine but also in the way that yoga in often practiced in the West, it is somehow limited only – or mostly – to the point of view of the physical body. Many people do not understand that if you can work at the level of the energy, the result – also at the level of the physical body, of the constituents, of the elements, and so on – is much more concrete and long lasting. If you ignore the function of the breathing or fail to understand its importance in the practice of yoga, you miss out on a major part of this knowledge. It is also true, as Doctor Phuntsog said, that if you exaggerate or do something in a wrong way, precisely because the function is so deep what can manifest is somehow a bigger problem.

For example, I went to teach in quite a well-known center in the USA where they have all these forms that you have to fill in and sign when you accept to teach there. One of the points was: "If you plan to teach anything related to techniques of breathing, please contact the director of the center first and discuss it with him." This is because breathing techniques are all also related with the emotional aspect of the mind, and that means these technique can potentially increase certain emotions. It is advised not to do certain more essential or powerful practices of breathing if you are in a state of anger or agitation. So, there is this aspect. However it is exactly this aspect that, when you know how to coordinate and use this function, makes it so important and so useful.

For example, the practice of Yantra Yoga is a sequence of movements. There are not many static positions that you have to try to find a way to hold. The only moment when you stop the sequence of the movements is when you stop the breathing.

In a way the essence of the practice of Yantra is designed around different kinds of holding. Different ways of holding the breath have different functions also regarding the five aspects of the wind that Doctor Phuntsog was describing. So, when you are able to coordinate this deeper aspect it is much more than just trying to make the body a little more toned and a little more flexible. It is not even necessary that you do very complicated and difficult things. You do not have to force, you just have to try to coordinate your capacity and condition in that moment.

So, the sequence of movements is related to inhaling, exhaling, and holding. And if you practice Yantra Yoga for a while, you can really directly experience that by relaxing and coordinating the breathing, the movement of the body becomes easier and more harmonious. It is as if the body becomes subtler, less tense. In reality you have to try to let go of tensions: without tensions you can be healthier, happier – this is another important aspect of the practice of Yantra Yoga – because our mind tends to be agitated. But if you use the wind element in the proper way, with the proper method, you can and you will relax the mind.

Of course, as Doctor Phuntsog said, if you really practice intensively it is better you remember that you have a physical body, that there is also the earth element that should be taken into account. For example, in some schools of *pranayama* in India even if they are vegetarian when they do intensive practice of *pranayama* they eat something nourishing like milk, butter, honey. So, you have to try to balance and coordinate all this. The system of Yantra Yoga itself works to coordinate all these different aspects, to harmonize our movements, harmonize our energy, harmonize our condition and therefore our health, our well-being.

When do you practice yoga? For example, recently in the USA there was a kind of uproar due to an article in the famous newspaper the *New York Times*, saying that by practicing yoga you can hurt yourself. Well, of course we still have a body, our energy, and mind, so it does not mean that if you practice yoga you suddenly enter into a paradise, just because you said the word yoga. So, if you force, if you are distracted, of course you can hurt yourself. You can hurt yourself cutting a tomato, so how is it possible you will not hurt yourself taking your foot and trying to push it where it does not want to go, without really understanding what you are doing. Forcing, either in quantity and quality, is not good. Ultimately you are the one who should try to understand your condition and do what is good for you without forcing. If you do that, if you can really coordinate different aspects, the practice of Yantra Yoga is fantastic, it is really incredible. It is important not to force, but also not to do anything: there should be a balance between being too active and being passive.

And the other aspect, as I said, is distraction. If you are distracted nothing works very well. You can have an accident with your car, you can cut your finger when you are cooking, and even if you do not hurt yourself you will not do a nice, correct, and fruitful practice of yoga. While if you are not distracted, if you stay with the breathing, relax into the breathing and you get rid of tensions the movement will follow and will be precise. Somehow you need to find a kind of natural balance.

In reality the practice of yoga is not to create something new, but just to eliminate the obstacles, just to get rid of what is hampering our condition. Natural is a wonderful word, but what does it really mean? When I teach Yantra Yoga sometimes we concentrate on the breathing. In Yantra Yoga we have to breathe completely from below up. When we refer to direct breathing, its means breathing through the nostrils, without being controlled or blocked or transformed. Most of the time there is an indication to breathe this way. Many people cannot do it. If you tell a person to breathe naturally, for this person breathing naturally is breathing unnaturally. So, the work of the practice is just to eliminate the tensions that do not allow you to breathe naturally according to your condition.

It is the same thing when we talk about alignment, which is a very important concept in yoga, but again, if you try to stick to a protocol of how the alignment should be, we are all different. When we practice Yantra or an *asana* we all try to do the same thing. For example, one position is called the Camel, and externally people seem to be doing it more or less the same way. But in reality everybody is doing his or her own Camel, because the body, energy, and mind of each person is in a different condition. But what is important is that there is this understanding and this presence and awareness that you do the best you can, with less tension and less effort, in the most harmonious way. Then it is perfect. A little more pushing forward, a little more arching backward, in that moment that is what is perfect.

But when you train, you can improve at different levels: you can improve your physical body; you can improve your flexibility, your capacity of breathing, and your capacity of relaxing the mind. In the end the ultimate purpose is really just to relax, to get rid of tensions and to be in this natural condition. So, in the end what we try to do is basically just to relax in this condition without tensions. It sounds nice, sounds simple, but is not always so simple. However, Yantra Yoga can be a good method to help you work in this direction. And then if you really want to understand and be stable in this condition then you have to follow a path, you have to follow a teacher. And that is basically what our Teacher teaches. So, the natural goal of Yantra Yoga is a spiritual teaching that Chögyal Namkhai Norbu is teaching.

I would like to finish here and leave some time for questions to Doctor Phuntsog or myself.

Q: What is the difference between Yantra Yoga and Shivananda?

A: Nowadays in the West several different traditions of Yoga have arrived. As far as I know, the first tradition that arrived was the tradition of Mongir, Shivananda. Some of the first Western teachers in Europe that spread knowledge of Yoga were Gerard Blitz and Andre Van Lisebeth. Then other schools that are now quite famous started to arrive: Ashtanga Yoga, Iyengar Yoga, Bikram Yoga, Vinyasa Yoga, and many others. What I recently heard is that there is a yoga done with weights. But what is peculiar to Yantra Yoga is a deep understanding and application of the function of the breathing and different kind of holdings of the breath coordinated with the movement and the rhythm. Just to be very simple, somehow, in general, breathing is sort of secondary in respect to the position, the *asana*. In Yantra Yoga it is the other way around. The position is like a servant of the breathing. The purpose of the position is to help shape a particular kind of breathing and holding.

Now there are other types of yoga in which the aspect of breathing is coordinated with the movement; there are also dynamic types of yoga. And in some instances some aspects of holding the breath are also applied, but never in the complete way that is the characteristic of Yantra Yoga, a system so complete and structurally articulated, dedicated to coordinating and harmonizing our energy by working at integrating and coordinating breathing and movement.

There is one interesting yoga sequence that is present in almost all the different systems of Yoga Schools, which is the Sun Salutation, or *suryanamaskara*. It is a series of movements coordinated with the breathing and, in some traditions includes a phase of holding. The real essence of yoga in all the ancient texts has always been the breathing as a fundamental bridge between the body and the mind. We cannot relax the mind if we do not coordinate our energy, and the breathing is the most powerful tool able to do it. This is the essence of the application of the principles of yoga.

But then, somehow, it became almost secondary. That is why I sometimes say that we have to go back to the future. We need to go back to the root of yoga to take it to the future. It looks like in the future the practice of yoga will become more and more focused on breathing. The ancient and precious tradition of Yantra Yoga can be very valuable knowledge on this journey. So, more or less, if you want to generalize, the difference is this.

For example, I had friends who practiced one school of yoga for ten or twelve years and still did not get any teachings of *pranayama*, the real *pranayama*, not just the one to change the air but the more complex, the deeper functioning. I myself was practicing Hatha Yoga – or what is called Hatha Yoga – and my interest for Yantra was the techniques of the breathing: deep, complex, complete techniques of the breathing. That is why I went the first time to receive this teaching. If you practice Yantra you can understand this, because before you really have the capacity to integrate breathing in the movement you have a taste of the practice, but when at a certain point you are able to do that, you experience that it is like a whole other thing. There is a different experience, a different quality.

Q: What is the reason, the root, of some respiratory illnesses?

A: When we look at the root of the breathing there can be four conditions creating imbalance: diet, behavior, seasonal influences, and provocations. The respiratory system is simply like a path or tube and when we talk about the three humors that I already explained, the phlegm humor is located in the chest area. It could be that this tube is blocked by the earth and water elements with condensed or sticky substances that generate asthma or difficulty in breathing.

The second cause may be that when we breathe we inhale a lot of impure air, which can cause the residue of impure breathing to accumulate in the breathing tube over a long time and cause problems. So, in simple words, one condition is combined with heat, one is combined or involved with a cold nature. The accumulation of a lot of mucus or congestion is part of the cold nature while having tensions in the chest region is more involved with heat. It can be the quality of breathing, as Fabio said, or the impure breathing.

Thank you for listening.

PRESENTATION

PHUNTSOG WANGMO
Diet, Behavior, and Care of Pregnant Women in Tibetan Medicine

January 13, morning (10:00)

Introduction

First of all, I would like to thank all the organizers for giving me this opportunity. As Chögyal Namkhai Norbu mentioned the other day, explaining Tibetan culture is not only in the interest of the Tibetan people or of myself; it is something that can be useful for all sentient beings. Of course, as a Tibetan, I do have, or I do feel I have, the responsibility of taking care of my culture and its knowledge, both by preserving it and by promoting it in the world. For that reason for about twenty years I have been working under the leadership of Chögyal Namkhai Norbu and following in his footsteps, trying to promote and preserve Tibetan culture. Therefore, as was said in the introduction, the Shang Shung Institute has established a Tibetan Medical School which was opened in 2005 at Tsegyalgar in Conway, Massachusetts. It is supported by the Dzogchen Community of Tsegyalgar and North America. This year we are going to open a second Tibetan Medical School at Kunsangar North in Russia. Of course, for this too we need the support of the International Community and especially the Russian Dzogchen Community.

When I say that I am trying to promote or preserve Tibetan culture, it does not mean I can do something by myself; it means I am following Chögyal Namkhai Norbu's example and his wishes. As he is our spiritual and cultural leader, he is everything for us. As a team, we follow his example and try to promote or preserve Tibetan culture and what that may mean. At this time, with the support and tireless work of the Barcelona and the Tenerife Dzogchen Communities together with the people of the International Community, we have this good opportunity to once again present Tibetan culture here in Tenerife. Even if we have a good leadership and a great culture to present to the world, without their support and collaboration it would be impossible for anything to manifest. So, on behalf of all the Shang Shung team, I take this opportunity to thank the organizers, the Barcelona Community, the Gakyil of Tenerife, the Gakyil of Barcelona, and the team that worked on this Tibetan event.

The Three Stages of Pregnancy

My topic today is how to take care of pregnant women. Everybody understands that this very important. Why? Because at some time we have all been in our mother's womb and in the future our generations will also come from the mother's womb. No one discusses how children come; that is the only way, in the past, present, and ideally also in the future.

The period of pregnancy is divided into three stages. The first is about how to conceive, when to conceive, and the necessary conditions for conception. The second phase concerns how the fetus develops in the mother's womb. The third concerns the signs or symptoms of birth and, once birth has occurred, how to take care of the baby.

First Stage: Conception

We all know that in order to conceive two main substances are needed: the father's sperm and the mother's egg. Everybody knows and accepts this. In Tibetan medicine and in Tibetan Buddhism these two are not sufficient to form a baby; we need a third, important, component that we call the consciousness.

Once it is a physically possible time and these three factors – the father's sperm, the mother's egg, and the consciousness – are ready to become linked together, then there is the *possibility* to conceive. In Tibetan medicine we say that first you need to have the cause for conceiving, then you have the action of conceiving, plus you have the karma; once you have all three together, cause, action, and karma, now there is a fruit.

For example, if we want to plant a flower, first we need the seed, then the soil, then we need other elements, plus the temperature must be perfect, and also we must work on that; then we have the possibility of the flower. We can have a lot of interesting seeds and good fertile soil, but if we do not work on it or put energy into it nothing will grow; we know that very well.

Of the three factors necessary for conception – sperm, egg, and consciousness – the first two are inseparable from the five elements; they are based on the five elements. The consciousness is not on the material level so we cannot say it is composed of the five elements, but it is supported by them: not the rough five elements, but the subtle ones. The consciousness needs to move on and is determined to find a family. In order to be able to move on and to determine the next life there must be a kind of energy, which is that of the five subtle elements.

In general, because all phenomena are composed of outer, inner, and the secret aspects, the five elements can be presented at three levels: the rough level that we can see, something that is visible; the more subtle level that we can feel or think about; and the very subtle level that we cannot even feel or think about. It is like the explanation of the mandala. There are various types of mandalas with different deities, but the idea of all mandalas is basically the same. They too have three aspects: outer, inner, and secret. The secret mandala means the center, like the heart. Our body can be described in a similar way: the outer structure of our body is the outer mandala; our organs are the inner mandala; and the center of the heart, or heart blood, is our secret mandala.

That is how it is explained in the medical texts. Yoga practice explains in a more subtle and deeper way. This also means that Tibetan medicine is not only a science of healing; Tibetan medicine is very developed both in the physical, visible aspects and in the inner, invisible energies. For this reason, its benefit does not come from any one herb or treatment; it maintains, balances, and treats the whole of the outer, inner, and secret body or the outer, inner, and secret elements. A different treatment is needed for each step.

As I said before, three components are needed in order to conceive: two of them are composed of the five elements and then the consciousness is supported by the five elements.

Once conception has occurred there are different symptoms we can observe. In general, a female is capable of conceiving from about twelve years old, or once the menstrual cycle starts, until around the fifties, that is to say during the time of the menstruation. The younger she is the better because she is healthier. We all know this. Why is it that we do not menstruate before twelve and after fifty? Before twelve the body needs to build muscles, blood, fat, bones, bone marrow, and the reproductive fluid. It needs to build them step by step. The reproductive fluid is the last of the seven body constituents to develop. Firstly we need the other components to be sufficiently developed in order to have a good enough substance to menstruate and to conceive.

We can think of a metaphor: when you graduate from school and just get a simple, small job, at that time you do not have enough money to go to parties or go on vacation because the money you make is just enough to pay for your food and other necessities. Jobs are usually paid very little when we have no experience. Similarly, what the body produces before twelve is just enough to build it; there is no extra substance for menstruation and conception.

And then from the age of about twelve until the fifties, for about thirty-eight years, there is menstruation. This means that now there is extra body substance to come out. After fifty the menstruation cycle stops. Why? Because all the organs, like machines, have declined and become older. Again they produce just enough to maintain the body but do not produce extra. With another metaphor you can simply think that, after retiring, your pension is just enough to pay for your living costs, there is no extra for going on vacation or having a fancy life. What I am saying is that in the midlife period a woman's body produce extra and in the first and third parts it produces less.

For men it is a little different. In Tibetan medicine the chapter on behavior says that until eighteen years old it is better for males not to have intercourse because, if they do, the pure part of the reproductive fluid transforms into the life-sustaining liquid, which we call *thigle*. Until eighteen years old this life-sustaining liquid or *thigle* is not well built and if you lose it, it is then a little hard to rebuild that substance.

Also in certain parts of the four seasons there is a limitation on intercourse because if you lose more reproductive fluid, or ejaculate during those times it causes loss of the essential *thigle*. When Doctor Kunchok presents the seasonal diet and the seasonal behavior, he will cover these things. For men there is obviously no menopause, so in comparison to women the period of fertility lasts longer.

The fact that women are usually fertile for about thirty-eight years does not mean that they can always conceive during that time. If sperm and egg are healthy then it is possible to conceive, but of course many problems can also occur. There are four causes that prevent conception (I am talking about physical problems): if either the sperm or the egg is contaminated by a wind [*lung*] disturbance; or if they are affected by *tripa*, which is the fire element; or affected by the phlegm element, which is a combination of earth and water; or by provocations. Any of these can prevent conception, due to physical causes.

All four can be treated. For example, if you have a wind element disturbance, or a fire element disturbance, both of them dry the seed so it is not sufficient for conception. Wind dries because its nature is rough; fire dries because it is heat. The result is the same; both make the substances insufficient. If the combination of earth and water elements – the phlegm – affects [the seed], then there is too much in quantity, but it is also too heavy, like mud; so it is not able to remain there, it is not able to produce growth; maybe it can conceive but it does not stay and cannot plant the fruit. But this condition can still be treated. If provocation affects [the seed], conception can be prevented in many ways. The symptoms of provocation are mysterious, there are no determined symptoms; many different kinds can manifest.

These are the physical impediments, but there are not only the physical causes, there are also karmic causes that can make conception possible or not. From the Buddhist point of view this is another topic. Anyway, when you conceive, there is a father, a mother, and something conceived, a fetus. This is not something accidental. Many young people think, "Oh, I didn't want a child; I conceived by accident." But it is not accidental; it is a karmic link.

Second Stage: Health Care During the Development of the Fetus

How do we need to take care once conception has occurred? That is my second topic, how we develop. To know how to take care we also need to know how to develop. When we plant a flower, if you ask me how you should take care, then first we need to know how to grow that flower. During the different stages of development from the planting of the seed until we get the fruit there is not only one way of taking care of the flower; each period has a different kind of taking care. For this reason we need to discuss a little bit how the fetus develops in the womb.

In Tibetan medicine we say pregnancy lasts thirty-eight weeks, which is nine months and ten days; in Western medicine they say it lasts forty weeks. But I think that basically the system of counting is the same. It depends on when conception happens during the menstruation cycle. In which period of time during the menstruation cycle can we conceive? In Tibetan medicine we say this possibility exists starting from the third day; also in Western medicine they say that it is possible to ovulate after you finish your menstruation cycle. One does not conceive during menstruation, one conceives after the bleeding has stopped. When the egg moves, when it comes down that is the time to conceive.

How does one know that one has conceived? In the woman the heartbeats are a little faster, she becomes a little weak, she looks tired: these are the first signs of having conceived. In the sutras it is said that the father feels the same, but in the mother the signs are more noticeable. In each week for thirty-eight weeks a wind comes. Then slowly, slowly the fetus develops.

The Stage of the Fish

In the first week the fetus is still like milk mixed with yogurt. In the second week that mixture of milk and yogurt assumes sort of an egg shape, a little oval shape. In the third week it becomes like yogurt. Starting that way till the second month the form is stable but the body is still liquid.

In the second month especially the shoulders and then the hips develop. This period is called the period of the fish. It means that the body is basically formed but the shoulders and hips are not yet strong or protruded, so during this period there is still a danger of miscarriage. In the first month this danger is greater because the fetus is liquid just like yogurt, the hardest part of it is like yogurt. In the second month it is more solid but still does not have hips and shoulders so there is nothing to block it; it is still like a fish, slippery, so it is easy to lose it. If you already have a history of miscarriage you need to be very careful during the first three months.

When the fourth week comes, the fetus is establishing its gender, either male or female. At that time the mother becomes a little emotionally unstable; it is easy for her to cry or to get angry. Her lower back especially becomes sort of heavy and painful. Also she desires to eat many tastes, including sour tastes. Why does the mother feel like eating many different tastes? That is not the desire of the mother but the desire of the fetus. During the time the fetus is forming its gender it has the strongest sort of desires, either male kinds of desires or female kinds.

So, even if a certain food is not healthy for the mother, you should mix it with some other food and give it to her because this is the desire of the fetus. For example, if the mother has high blood pressure, or weakness of the kidney, or the heartbeat is not regular, during pregnancy the blood pressure goes up. In case the mother has a desire for salty tasting food – you know that normally salt is not good for high blood pressure – you mix it with some other food. For example, when you make bread you add salt to the dough; then you can give it to her. This is because flour and wheat products have a sweet taste. If the mother has a kidney problem or indigestion problems but still likes to eat a lot of wheat products, like pasta, maybe that is the desire of the fetus. So we can give it to the mother, she can have pasta or wheat products if they are mixed with some cardamom or nutmeg, something warm, spicy.

To put it simply, she should have everything her body desires, even if you think it is not good for her health, but it should be mixed with something good. This can help. If we do not give it to her, what happens? We say that the fetus is unsatisfied and once the baby is born, he has symptoms of dissatisfaction, he always feels some unhappiness inside. During this time the mother has nausea, and maybe vomits; she has all the symptoms we call morning sickness, pregnancy sickness.

The Stage of the Turtle

Starting from then until the fifth month the body, organs, and limbs of the fetus develop. I am not saying that head and limbs do not appear until that moment; they appeared at the beginning, but now they are more visible. Also the arms and legs have grown. It means that the baby is growing bigger, pushing out from the mother's umbilicus, so the mother's abdomen protrudes. The limbs are growing and the fetus is starting to move inside the belly.

We call this the stage of the turtle. In that period there is less danger of miscarriage, but in case something happens it is more dangerous for the mother's life than in the first three months. If something happens in the first three months the shoulders of the baby are still not grown, so it is easier to lose it, easier for it to come out. But in the second period, in case the baby dies in the mother's womb or something happens, she would need to go to hospital and probably we would need to perform surgery to take it out.

While the baby is developing we should focus more on the mother, mainly on three things. Firstly, we try to see that the fetus develops well and is healthy; secondly, we try to prevent the increasing of the wind element in the mother, both at a physical and at a mental level; thirdly, we help her to have labor on time.

The first point means both maintaining the mother's good health and the development of the fetus, so it concerns food. If the mother is eating and developing the baby, basically one mouth is feeding two bodies, so she needs to eat more in quantity and in quality. In this case substantial food such as dairy products and meat products are good. These are good because they belong to the category of the sweet tastes.

Food has six basic tastes, each with its own potential or function or power. They are: sweet, sour, salty, bitter, hot, and astringent. Why do we have six different tastes and functions? Each taste has two predominant elements. The sweet taste has a predominance of earth and water elements; the sour taste has fire and earth elements; the salty taste has fire with water elements; the bitter taste has wind and water elements; the hot taste has wind and fire elements; the astringent taste has earth and wind elements. These six tastes are a combination of or have a predominance of two elements. This does not mean that the other elements are not present. When we want to grow something all five elements are needed, but some of them are more predominant, some less predominant or less in quantity. The result is different tastes and different functions. During pregnancy, when the mother is feeding the baby, the sweet taste is good, the sour taste is good; also the salty taste is fine. Bitter is not good; hot is not good; astringent is also not that good. Why? Because hot is made of the fire and wind elements and both are drying. We do not need to dry, we need to develop, to make bigger, we need to build, not to shrink, and dry means that it becomes smaller and shrinks, no? Even if the mother is a little big and wants to lose weight, for the purpose of the fetus in this moment it is not good to go on a diet, like a vegetarian diet or a raw-vegetable diet, or others. It is not the best moment, because she needs to build.

The second point is that mentally and physically the mother needs to keep calm. In this case oil treatment is important, it is very good in many ways. In fact, when women get pregnant it is very good and happy news, a very enjoyable moment, but at the same time physically and emotionally there is also a big responsibility. In general, samsara is always something to worry about; that is nothing new. But for a woman her first worry is to conceive; then once she has conceived, it is how the baby develops in the womb and then how she can give birth. That is a huge transition. Then she is worried about the baby. When the baby grows up and so forth, she has endless worries. She is worried not only mentally, but also physically she has a big responsibility.

One of the elements more involved during pregnancy is the wind element. Why? The wind element is located in the lower part of the body. In terms of the three poisons, it is a symbol of attachment. Attachment is located in the lower part of the body. Attachment is the symbol of desire. One of the winds, which is called the descending wind, is located in the pelvic region. One of its major functions or jobs is closing and opening the "gates." During pregnancy, for many reasons, either because of physical problems or mental worries, this wind goes up. The nature of wind is very rough; the nature of wind is very subtle; the nature of wind is very unstable. Simply, if you think of a very active person she behaves like a three-year old child: if you have a three-year old child you need to pay careful attention to her; you cannot lose sight of her. It is the same with the wind nature; you need to pay attention to it.

What happens if the wind goes up or down, which means that you either get a lot of wind or a deficiency of wind? It can cause a premature birth or, when the time comes, a delayed birth, also causing the overdevelopment of the fetus in the mother's womb.

For these reasons oil massage is very good because its nature is smooth. We put oil on our body when we have dry skin, because it is the antidote to wind, to dryness. You heat up the oil, making it extra warm but without boiling it. That is also very important. You can use it on the entire body, but there are three special points where you can use it. One is the lower back, the sacrum area. Why? Firstly it is because the sacrum region is the main location of wind. Wind is light and rough, oil is heavy and smooth, so oil counteracts the wind and makes it calm down. Secondly, we want to move the joints: without lubrication our joints make a creaking sound and get inflammation, we know this. Lubrication has the nature of phlegm, which is a combination of the earth and water elements. Without heat, the earth and water elements together are like mud, they are dull, not moving, sleeping. Therefore a warm oil compress reduces the coolness and heats up, so when the labor time comes it is easier for the joints to move. If the joints move better, they can open wider, then the baby can come out in smoother and easier way.

Another part of the body to massage with oil is the inner thighs. One of the pathways of wind is via the inner thighs, so massaging there is also very important. It is close to the lower "gate," which is like a main entrance, and is also part of the desire region, so it is important to do oil massage there. Its purpose is both to prevent wind problems and to promote a smooth labor. Another important zone is the abdomen. It is good for the wind to give a little oil massage to the tummy. It also especially prevents stretch marks, the scars that usually appear on the skin during pregnancy. In simple words, during pregnancy it is important to eat good food, do oil massage, and try to keep the mother happy.

The Stage of the Pig

The period between the fifth and the seventh month is called "the stage of the pig." This means that now the baby is totally developed, not in the sense that he is big but that everything is formed. He is eating from the mother, living within a tiny room, eating and sleeping, so we call that the stage of the pig.

Again it is very important to eat good food because the baby is already formed but still needs to develop and grow bigger. At this time the mother's diet is not specifically focused on the three tastes (sweet, sour, and salty); in this second part it is a combination, there is a need for more variety of food. The reason is that if the baby grows too big in the mother's womb, it is dangerous for the baby and for the mother when the labor comes. So, in this period a combination of sweet, astringent, and some sour tastes is good. It is also very important for the mother's diet to add some spices to make food lighter. Today there is not enough time to discuss all the natures of food, but the chapter on diet is a very comprehensive subject in Tibetan medicine. To give the example of barley: barley has its taste, its functions, and its nature. But then, the quality of barley is also affected by when it is harvested. And depending on the region the barley comes from – if it is desert, middle climate, or near the ocean, near the water – it has a different nature. Also depending on how you prepare it, if you cook it like a *tsampa* soup or you knead it like *tsampa* dough, it has also a different nature. So Tibetan diet is a huge topic; when we teach it in school it takes a whole semester, so we cannot cover it now. Anyway the astringent, sweet, and sour tastes are good in that period.

When the seventh month comes the baby is growing bigger. At that time he has a good memory of his past lives and again the mother is more emotional: for instance, she cries and laughs more easily. During this time the baby has memories of the past. Then, while growing, the memories slowly, slowly fade, like when you put new information into a computer and it deletes old information because there is not enough space. That is why today we do not remember anything of past lives, which is maybe a good thing.

Starting from the thirty-sixth to the thirty-seventh week the baby begins to think he or she wants to escape from that place because he feels it is very small, sticky, stinky, dark, and wet. He does not want to stay there; he wants to go away somehow. Until that point the baby found it was a very calm, warm, quiet place.

When explaining how the consciousness enters the mother's womb, we say that some consciousnesses know where they are going and some do not know, they are confused when entering. It looks like an open place with strong wind and rain and everybody looking for a shelter. Then somehow they enter, but do not know where they are entering. This confused way of entering is common for the majority of the people. Some know they are entering into the mother's womb, but there is not the feeling or idea that, "This is my place, this is my path, where I want to go." Only very few, extraordinary people or, in simple words, I would say, "reincarnated" people know where they are going. Anyway, both kinds enter into the mother's womb because they want to find a quiet, warm, happy, safe place. But when the thirty-sixth to the thirty-seventh week comes, they no longer like to stay there; they try to look for another place. So slowly, slowly the fetus looks for a gate where he can exit and slowly, slowly turns the head down toward the lower gate.

The Third Stage: Birth

The third part of our topic concerns the birth. When the baby is turning its head downward searching for the gate, the mother is having the signs or symptoms of the labor. The symptoms occur in her dreams, in her physical body, and in her emotions.

Her physical body becomes weaker; she gets lazy, and she gets heavier, especially in the lower part of her body. Her genital region also becomes heavier and enlarges. Emotionally she has more anxiety and fear because this is a huge responsibility. It can be joyful to have a beautiful baby but, unfortunately, also something unexpected can happen.

Today, in modern society, this part of medicine has developed well, so giving birth is safer. But before I came to the Western countries I was working in my country, East Tibet. I was the only doctor in the region, so every day I was attending to a minimum of fifty patients. From morning to twelve in the evening there was always something to do and sometimes they were unexpected things like helping a woman give birth. That was really a tough responsibility. Sometimes women were living on the mountains and it was difficult to get there. Also for the mother it was difficult to go down to the doctor because the time was very limited. Humans can be very elegant, they can look very strong, but once the breath stops they are gone. Even if you are famous, or beautiful or wealthy, no matter what you are, when you stop breathing life is finished. So I had a hard time in eastern Tibet when I was working with mothers and children.

An expectant mother can have indications in dreams of whether she is going to have a boy or girl. If she is wearing white clothes, or dancing, or singing, she is likely to have a boy; if she is wearing red-colored ornaments, like jewelry, or singing and talking or enjoying with a man, she is more likely to have a girl.

Anyway, when we have the signs of the birth time, traditionally we need two preparations. One is a sort of welcoming the baby, a sort of tradition; the other is the medical part: how we prevent danger for the mother and the child.

As regards the medical part, once the mother has given birth there can be many dangers, but if it is a natural birth, we need to prevent the bleeding and to keep the winds from going up, because while giving birth the cervix of the womb is open, so the wind goes up very much. It is also a big transition, so the wind goes up again. She is losing either a lot or a small quantity of blood, and that also causes the wind to go up. That is why we need to prepare certain kinds of food for the mother, like meat broth, or bone soup, or roasted barley flour, which we call *tsampa*, cooked in milk. This means it is nutritious food, but it is not cool or heavy, it is light and easy to digest.

At the same time we work on the wind points. After giving birth, the upper wind points are more important while during pregnancy the lower wind points are more important. During labor, some injuries, like wounds could have happened inside the womb; for this reason it is very important to prevent infections. Also sometimes some bits of placenta or small parts of tissue remain inside, which can later cause infection. For this reason traditionally we give a medicine called *zhije chucig*, the main ingredient of which is rhubarb. Rhubarb medicine cleans the uterus. There is also another medicine we make, based on lavender, which is very good for shrinking the uterus.

So, what I am saying is simply that after giving birth until the first month it is very important that women take warm, nutritious food. The first three tastes, sweet, sour, and salty are more nutritious. The first six months the baby is getting food from the mother's milk, breastfeeding. This is again like one mouth feeding two bodies; therefore it is important to have the first three tastes. After six months the baby starts eating, so you can start to introduce solid food.

When a baby is born there are traditionally three welcomes. One is the welcome for joining the samsara or the new family. First we wash the baby in half water and half milk. There are two reasons for putting in the milk. One is that milk is creamy, so it keeps the baby's skin smooth. For nine months the baby was in his mother's womb, in a sort of lubrication, of water; once he gets into our hands they are too rough for him; the milk softens our touch, so it does not feel too rough. Another reason is that milk is the essence nutrition from the cow, so it is a very nutritious food; it is also white and is a non-violent product so it is like a symbol for the white path.

Secondly, we put a small bracelet of garlic on him because it protects him from provocations. In fact in childhood it is very dangerous to be attacked by provocations.

Thirdly, we also symbolically write the Manjushri mantra on the baby's tongue out of the wish that his speech be good and wise.

This is how traditionally we take care of mother and child in Tibetan medicine and culture.

PRESENTATION

LHUSHAM GYAL
Methods of Diagnosis

January 13, morning (11:30)

Greetings to everyone. Today I would like to talk about diagnosis.

In Tibetan medicine the topic of diagnosis is thought of as having two parts: the first part is the content of the diagnosis, the principles and the theory of how to diagnose. The second part concerns the actual practical methods used, that is to say asking questions, looking or inspecting, and also touching.

The content part of diagnosis, or principal theory, has three sections: one deals with how to diagnose different types of patient. Since each patient has a different psychological belief and understanding, physicians look at the situation according to the patient and then make a diagnosis. The methods part concerns techniques for making a good diagnosis, based on the methods used by doctors.

Questioning Method
As we said, the actual methods involve looking, touching, and also questioning. Touching basically refers to pulse reading, while looking concerns urine analysis, both of which are unique to Tibetan medicine. The third skill, which is the questioning method, the anamnesis, is

more common as it is also used in Western medicine. As a background of the investigative method, the questioning method, usually we ask the patient about the causes of his illness. We ask about a number of factors, details of the patient's life history, and particularly details of behavior and diet, and so on. Sometimes, for example, a particular problem may be caused by some particular food or drink. So we try to discover this by asking many questions. As a qualified doctor in Tibet the questioning diagnosis also includes asking the patient about their natural pulse. This is because in traditional Tibetan society when a child is eight years old, a qualified doctor is asked to identify the nature of the child's pulse, for example whether it is *potsa*, or male pulse, *motsa*, or female pulse, or *changchub semtsa*, a neutral pulse; these are the three kinds of pulse nature. And then another factor is the nature of the person, whether it is *lung* or *tripa* or *pekan*. So this too will be asked as part of the anamnesis. If the society is not familiar with this kind of Tibetan medicine it will be more difficult, but these indications provide a kind of general background information. That is traditionally how people practice in Tibet.

If the situation has not been brought out through questioning sometimes misdiagnosis can occur. For example, for people with the *motsa* pulse, which is one of the three types of pulse, if the patient does not know his natural pulse, then maybe the doctor may risk misdiagnosing it, classifying him as having a *tripa* disorder, [because both the *motsa* and *tripa* pulses tend to be fast and thin].

So it is very important to ask questions before reading the pulse or carrying out the urine analysis because Tibetan medicine also emphasizes that reading a pulse without having particular knowledge can sometimes be very difficult. Therefore, you have to ask good questions to discover what the situation is. Sometimes it is very difficult because patients are not always honest with their doctor, some do not say anything, then the doctor has to find out what the problem is just by reading the pulse and if he only has that to go by, he needs to be a really good doctor.

Visual Examination

The second method is to visually examine the patient. This includes examining the patient's eyes: eye color and the pattern of the nerve system in the eyes; examining the tongue, including its color; the facial skin tone; and also the urine, the blood, the sputum, the vomit, all of these can be examined visually by the physician.

When examining the eyes, for instance, sometimes they can be yellow around the eyeball: that is considered sign of a *tripa* disorder, which means there is more heat in the body. And sometimes the person cannot concentrate with the eyes, cannot look at things in a concentrated way: that is probably sign of a *lung* disorder. And sometimes red around the rims of the eyeballs can mean increased blood pressure.

For example, looking at the sputum, if there is coughing that produces sputum and the spit is bubblier it is a sign of a *lung* disorder. If the spit is more salty and kind of white, it indicates a disorder of heat and lungs.

In the case of vomit, if it is more like raw food, this is undigested food coming out, which will be diagnosed as weak digestion and a stomach problem. If the vomit is sour, it is diagnosed as the early stage of *pekan mugpo*, which is more a syndrome of the digestive system particularly in the stomach. These are some examples of simple inspection diagnosis.

Tongue Diagnosis

Tongue diagnosis and urine analysis are particularly important, so I will explain them in more detail.

In tongue examination, if the person is healthy the color of the tongue is more red and also more soft, it has more saliva, it is more flexible. Those are considered signs of a normal person. If it is the opposite then the person might have any number of disorders. In a *lung* disorder the tongue will be dry, very red and very rough. In a *pekan* disorder usually the color of the tongue is not particularly identified with one color, it is more whitish and will have a thick white coating on the surface. In a *tripa* disorder the tongue will be more yellow. On the surface of the tongue the coating will be more yellow. So there is a kind of yellow color in the tongue. If someone has heart disease, meaning they are stressed out or suffer from anxiety, the person's tongue will be red and dry. More importantly the root of the tongue is dark and on the surface of the tongue there is often a split, a cut.

Urine Analysis

Urine analysis is a visual and objective diagnosis, so it is easier for physicians to use because there are things you can see from the urine, it is like looking in a mirror. It is easier than pulse reading.

Urine analysis involves several different steps. The first one is the preparation. To be able to examine the real, original color or nature of the urine, preparation is very important. The color of urine is affected by diet, food, and drink, so the patient must not take food that colors the urine, like vitamins or strong food because they alter the color of the urine. If the person drinks alcohol the elements of the body will be different. The patient needs to show the real symptoms of any disorders he might have, not as affected by strong foods or alcohol, for example. You also need to be careful of lifestyle and behavior. For example, if you need to have a urine test, you should not go swimming the day before, or do much exercise, or sit in the sun too long. These activities need to be avoided otherwise the urine will be affected.

Then the time for the urine examination is also very precise. Usually the urine sample is taken in the morning, so the evening before the person should not eat or drink strong food but normal food and then in the early morning, the first time the person urinates he or she should discard the first portion of urine and collect only the middle stream. These urine samples will show very precisely the situation in the person's body. The container used to collect the urine must be white; it cannot be dark or any different colors because the physician needs to look at the urine in order to see the color of the froth or the natural color.

So all this is the preparation. Once the preparation has been carried out precisely we need to examine the urine. We look at the urine three times after the urine sample is taken, and there are nine steps to follow for inspecting urine.

As regards the time to look at the urine sample, one is right after taking the urine sample, which is "the time of the heat," because the urine is still warm. During that time there are four things to look at: the color, any cloudiness, the smell, and the froth. So in investigating the nature of the urine you can look at the color of the urine and also look at any cloudiness. Sometimes the physician smells the urine, the smell can be strong or weak or mild. And then sometimes a good doctor will even inspect the taste as well, what kind of taste the urine has. These are also part of the method of inspecting urine.

The second time is called the "lukewarm time." During this time we look at two things: one is the sediment, to see if there is some deposit like sand or dust in the urine. Then second is the cream, which is the top of the urine: there may be some kind of creamy film on the surface of the urine.

The third time is the "cold time." So, the urine sample is kept for a while and then becomes cold. During the cold time you can look at three things: firstly, the way the nature itself of the urine has changed, if the change was fast or slow. Then the second thing is the specific urine changes: if it changed from the bottom of the container or from the sides or from the surface. Then thirdly after the urine changed, we examine whether the urine is still light or dusty or very dirty, i.e., the appearance of the urine.

These are the precise steps as they are described in the textbooks, three different times and nine things to look at in the urine. This is the normal method of diagnosis. When the urine is brought from far away, usually it is put on a fire to boil or keep warm and then examined in the three stages of the urine diagnosis. That is the general background of how we use our knowledge to diagnose urine.

Urine of a Healthy Person

Now I would like to talk about the kind of urine a normal person has. A normal person's urine color is a mixture of white and yellow; we usually use the example of melted butter. The color of the urine is similar to boiled or cooked butter. And the smell is not so strong, it is a mild smell. And then when you stir it with a stick to look at the froth, the bubbles are neither big nor too small, they are more medium size. During the lukewarm time in a normal person's urine, the sediment is also very, very light, sometimes even hard to see. And the cream on the surface of the urine is very thin, very, very light. During the cold time the nature of the urine changes. It changes from the sides. It means that in the container its nature changes from all around the sides and becomes very light, like water, and its color is very light, like a mixture of white and yellow. That is for a normal healthy person's urine. Then you need learn the signs of disordered urine. The disorders depend on a variety of illnesses and therefore are more complex.

Disordered Urine

For disorders, we first learn about normal urine. Then with that as our baseline, in a *lung* disorder the urine will be more bluish in color. If the color is more whitish it is a *pekan* disorder. If it is yellowish it is more of a *tripa* disorder. So that is how we can identify by the color.

If the urine sample is very cloudy it means that the body has the nature of a heat problem, a *tshawa* disorder. Sometimes the cloudiness lasts, it does not disappear quickly, so that is more like a hidden *tshawa* disorder, meaning a heat or hot disorder. If the cloudiness is minimal and not very thick, that is more *drangwa*, a cold disorder. That, then, is a brief summary of urine analysis in Tibetan medicine.

In terms of precise diagnosis for each disorder or disease there is a lot of content, which we have not enough time to cover today. So these are just some examples for you to understand. This kind of urine diagnosis is unique in the traditions of medicine. Many researchers have studied that Tibetan medicine has this complex understanding and theory of urine analysis. Some scholars have also said that there might be some relationship with ancient Roman traditional medicine. We do not know whether there are such connections or not, but what *is* true is that this urine analysis is a very complex study in Tibetan medicine.

Pulse Reading

The last technique is the palpation diagnosis: the doctor can touch any part of the body to look at any disorder or problem. But in Tibetan traditional medicine reading a pulse is the most unique so I would like to talk a little bit more about that.

Pulse reading has similar requirements to urine analysis, for example the preparation. When the patient needs to have a pulse reading, the day before he must not do any strenuous activities and also needs to observe some dietary guidelines. In urine analysis it is more important to be careful with food because the color of the urine would be affected. But for the preparation or prerequisites of pulse reading, behavior or lifestyle is more important because the nature of the pulse will be changed by certain extreme behaviors. The best time for reading the pulse is usually in the morning. As in Tibet the family physicians and doctors mostly go to the patients' house to examine them, then so that the energy inside the room is not dispersed, the patient just gets up and remains warm inside the house. The patient does not eat or take any coffee or any food or drink, and the physician will read his pulse just before breakfast. That is the best time.

The second factor to consider is the location of the pulse reading. Usually in the textbooks it says starting two fingers from the first wrinkle on the wrist, three fingers are put there: *tshon, kan, chag,* or index, middle finger, and ring finger. So, three fingers are used at the place of the pulse on both the left and right wrist to look at the major five solid organs and six hollow organs. Two things need to be considered in the pulse. One is the overall, general nature of the pulse: the pulse can be higher or lower, or tight or loose, or it can beat faster or slower. Secondly one has to look at the lungs, heart, liver, at all the major organs precisely.

How precisely does the physician take the pulse of a patient? For example, when checking the pulse of a male, the upper part of the index finger feels the heart pulse; the lower part feels the heart and intestine. The middle finger feels the pulse for the spleen and stomach; the ring finger senses the left kidney and spleen. So the upper part of a finger sounds out the major organs and the lower part sounds out the hollow organs.

The pulse reading is very complicated. It is very hard for beginners to learn right away, so this is just a simple introduction. Usually what they do is first learn the nature of the pulse. There are twelve different natures: for example, the pulse can be tight or loose, faster or slower, or higher or lower. You need to understand these first and then gradually learn to understand more, for example the liver pulse versus the heart pulse, and so on.

With the left hand, under the upper part the of index finger the physician feels the pulse for the lungs and under the lower part for the large intestine. Under the middle finger, the upper part senses the liver and the lower part the gallbladder. And under the ring finger, the upper part tunes into the left kidney and the lower part the urinary bladder. This is a very precise knowledge and wisdom. Each finger senses two major organ pulses. Usually the upper parts of the fingers feel the major organs and the lower parts feel the hollow organs. This is a very subtle and deep wisdom to understand.

Beginners usually start by examining the normal person's pulse. Once you understand a normal person's pulse – the pulse of a person who is not ill – it will be easier to examine an ill person's pulse. Usually we can divide everybody's pulse into three categories: *po*, or male; *mo*, or female; and *changchub semtsa*, a neutral pulse. But also different people can have very different natures of pulse. Sometimes the normal person's pulse can behave like a diseased person's pulse, and this needs to be identified precisely, otherwise it can be difficult to understand when the person is sick. For example, in a pregnant woman usually the pulse is very strong, it almost touches the doctor's fingers. Usually she would have a normal pulse beat, but it changes a little bit when she is pregnant. Through the pulse reading there are more particular things we can observe using specific methods. For example, it is possible to identify through the pulse whether a woman is carrying a female or a male fetus.

We also know that our bodies are connected with the external environment, like summer versus winter and spring versus fall for instance, and throughout the seasons the nature of the pulse will also change. So for a physician it is very important to learn these various changes or phenomena of the pulse.

One aspect of the method of reading the pulse is the pulse rate, or how many times the pulse beats. In Tibetan medicine in one inhalation and exhalation of a normal, healthy person, such as the physician, a pulse rate of five beats would be normal. This means the body is neither *tshawa* nor *drangwa*, it is neutral, it is very healthy. This kind of pulse rate matches with Western medicine; a pulse rate of 75 beats per minute matches this quite closely.

We have only explained what it should be for a normal person, maybe this kind of basic information is useful for you to understand just as a background. For an ill or disordered person actually it is very complex and obviously we do not have enough time. But very briefly it can be described as below.

Pulse Reading in a Sick Person

Usually a disorder or disease is called *ne* in Tibetan. *Nechen* means a person who has a *ne*, a sick person. Disorders can be divided into two categories: *tshawa* and *drangwa*. *Tshawa* is literally translated as heat or hot, while *drangwa* means cold-nature diseases. These two kinds of general categories are used in pulse reading.

There are twelve different types of pulses, six for *tshawa* disorders and six for *drangwa* disorders. The first type of pulses is strong for *tshawa* disorders and weak for *drangwa* disorders.

The second type is what we describe as "developed" for *tshawa* disorders: the pulse is full, you can feel it, it is more like coming to the surface of the skin. The corresponding pulse in *drangwa* disorders is more sunken or deep: you have to push your finger hard to find it.

The third type is "twisted" in *tshawa* disorders; when you touch it is almost jumping out at your fingers. The corresponding pulse in a *drangwa* disorder can be described as "depleted"; it is very hard to find.

And then the fourth type is fast for *tshawa* and slow for *drangwa*. For example, earlier we talked of a basic rate of five times during one breath, but if it beats maybe six times, seven times, that is *tshawa*, while three or four beats per breath cycle will be slow, indicating *drangwa*.

The fifth type is tight in *tshawa* disorders: when you push, inside the pulse feels like it is tightened. In a *drangwa* disorder, it is very loose, the opposite of tight.

Finally, the sixth type is very hard in *tshawa* disorders, like metal or steel, while in *drangwa* disorders it is described as "empty."

This is a very general overview. As a beginner you can identify these precise beating natures of the pulse and then later you can learn the others. Earlier we talked about how it is more normal for doctors to diagnose disorders of the health of the body and how situations of illness can be identified through pulse reading. But there are also more diagnoses. For example, people can look at the pulse on the top of the feet to tell how long the person may live. In the case of a very severely ill person, for example, we can read that pulse to diagnose how long the person has to live, when the person will die. And then another thing to look at in the pulse is the life strength of a person. That is called *latsa*. For such things we can use these techniques to look at the person's situation.

Because of the limited time we have to stop here. If you are interested more in diagnosis you should read more books and also attend seminars to learn more. We would like to have more lectures in the future and hope you will be able to learn more. Thank you very much.

PRESENTATION

KUNCHOK GYALTSEN
and PHUNTSOG WANGMO
Tibetan External Medicine, Theory and Demonstration

January 13, afternoon

Kunchok Gyaltsen

Good afternoon. I would like to give you a general introduction to the external therapies practiced in Tibetan medicine. Doctor Phuntsog will then explain what Kunye massage therapy is and our colleague Aldo Oneto will give a practical demonstration.

There are three aspects to Tibetan medicine. The first concerns the human body and mind and the various categories of illnesses in general. The second concerns diagnosis. The third concerns therapy or treatment.

Four lines of treatments are used: diet, behavior, medicine or herbs, and external therapies.

The Tibetan term for external is *che*. The literal meaning of *che* is analysis, but in this case we use palpation or our sense of touch to analyze what is wrong in the physical body and find out the problems. Then we use various techniques to take away the pain or illnesses or problems. That is the overall meaning of *che*. Many different therapy techniques exist in Tibetan medicine. However, the main textbook, called *Gyüzhi* or *Four Tantras*, names five kinds of external therapies.

The first is called *tug* in Tibetan, meaning to apply heat to certain points on the body. The second is *lum,* medicinal baths. The third is *chugpa,* which mainly includes Kunye. The fourth is *metsa*, or moxibustion. The last is *tharka*, which is translated as bloodletting.

Each of these five methods has a different purpose: bloodletting, or *tharka*, is for treating heat disorder, called *tsawa*. *Metsa*, moxibustion, is used for cold disorder, or *trangwa*. *Chugpa*, which is mostly Kunye therapy, is used for combinations of disorders involving *lung, tripa*, and *pekan*, especially where *lung* problems prevail. In *lung, tripa* and *pekan* combinations with a preponderance of *pekan* disorder, *tug* is used to heat certain points. In combinations of *lung, tripa*, and *pekan* where the main problem is with *tripa* disorders, we use *lum*, medicinal baths.

For *tug* therapy, doctors mostly use two kinds of methods. One is *drötug*, which involves applying heat to points. An example of *drötug* is *horme*, where herbs are wrapped in cotton fabric and then heated in butter and placed on the body points. For treating *tsawa* or heat disorders, stones and other objects are chilled and then placed on specific points.

Lum, the external therapy of medicinal baths, can be done in various ways. One is natural baths, for instance in a hot spring, in which case warm sand, or stones, or the heat of the sun can be used to warm the body. One can also use *tsi nga lum*, a compound made of five medicinal herbs: you make an infusion of the herbs and put it into the water. Then stay in the water taking the medicinal bath. The same medicine can also be used in steam. These kinds of compounds are called *chu mig lum*, meaning they are created by human beings, by doctors. There are many ways for physicians to make this kind of *chu lum*. These types of medicinal baths are usually very effective and the techniques are not difficult to use. They are particularly effective for arthritis and for people who live in humid areas.

Then we have the external therapy called *chugpa*, which as I said is mainly Kunye, using olive oil, medicinal oil, various other oils, or butter. Three steps are generally involved. The first one, *chug*, is to rub or press the body; the second is *nye*, making it softer; then the third is wiping the body. Doctor Phuntsog will explain more about Kunye later on.

As far as the external therapy of *metsa* or moxibustion is concerned, there are many different ways to apply it. Sage is burned and used to heat specific points. Sometimes the points are burned directly, sometimes they are heated indirectly, but there are many ways to do it and it is a very effective method.

And then the last external therapy is *tharka* or bloodletting. *Tharka* is very different from Western bloodletting. When we mention it Westerners and even Chinese people are often scared, because they think that bloodletting is a difficult treatment. But in Tibetan medicine, if someone needs to do *tharka*, they first need to take a medicinal decoction that divides the blood into impure blood and pure blood. Then the impure blood is bled from a certain point. During the bleeding, when you compare the impure blood and the pure blood you can see that the impure blood is dark and thick; it is very different. Only a very qualified and skilled doctor can do bloodletting, not everyone can do it; with *tharka* we need to be very careful. Skilled doctors using *tharka* look at the blood and can also identify further diseases, like diseases caused by evil spirits, for example. So it is a very useful and complex knowledge in Tibetan medicine; it is part of our tradition.

These are the five main external therapies in Tibetan medicine. They are mainly meant to be practiced by skillful and knowledgeable doctors. In fact, when you look at Kunye it seems like such a simple practice that anyone can do, but you must understand the circulation in the body of the energy called *la*, and also the factor of time, how the external universe communicates with the internal body. That is why astrology and astronomy are very important, and this is why in Tibetan we use the term *mantsi*: *man* means medicine and *tsi* means astronomy, astrology. So if people do not have knowledge of these four aspects it is very dangerous to do any kind of external therapy. Once you understand all these factors in an appropriate way, these become wonderful treatments and you can get rid of a lot of problems. So, it is very important to have this knowledge.

I will now hand over to Doctor Phuntsog.

Phuntsog Wangmo

The three of us are here today to present external therapies, and I am very happy to have this opportunity to present them to you. When we study external therapies in Tibetan medicine, the curriculum at school takes one long semester to complete, not just two hours. In the United States we teach Tibetan Kunye at the International Shang Shung Institute. The curriculum is a 750-hour course. So needless to say you will not be able to learn everything today and then apply it tomorrow. As a team, we will try to do our best to explain it to you based on our capacity.

There are two different ways to apply Kunye: on the floor and on the table. When we work on the floor we use a very thick mattress made with nice, natural materials, not something made of a plastic and then covered. Please do not expect that a Tibetan Kunye massage is performed on a cold, cement floor covered with rubber. Healing is an art, we call it an art.

When we receive a treatment there are many factors that make us feel better. One is the doctor or practitioner's warm welcome; kindness and a loving approach definitely help the patient feel better. Another factor is not only warmth and kindness on the part of the doctor but also the environment. Plus, of course, the doctor or practitioner's skill and the power of medicine and so forth are very important. Today's conference gives us a unique opportunity to demonstrate the practice to you in a simple way, so I will explain for about fifteen minutes what Kunye is, and then Aldo Oneto will demonstrate while I continue explaining.

Kunye is one of the traditional Tibetan treatments. It is not some kind of new age massage; this type of treatment has been practiced for thousands of years. *Ku* refers to applying oil on the body, while *nye*, as Doctor Kunchok said, is like rubbing to make the body smooth or soft. Why is Kunye a very helpful and common treatment? As we explained this morning and yesterday, our body functions through the five elements. These five elements are the foundation or base of our body as well as of the functions of our body. They are both the cause or condition of sickness or diseases and the key to treatment. So this is something truly unique to Tibetan medicine: everything is based on the five elements. This knowledge gives us a very good understanding of why we need to balance the elements, how we balance them, and what we are treating. Also, because it is based on that knowledge in Tibetan medicine we do not have such strong side effects. In general, anything that helps inevitably also harms. Anything that has positive effects has also negative effects. But Tibetan medicine does not have strong side effects. Why? Because we understand very well what the body is, what we are working on; so once we have a good understanding of our body, antidotes are also based on that nature, and as a consequence the side effects are minimal. In terms of the function of the five elements in the body, Kunye can be applied either in the case of wind nature, what we call *lung* imbalance, or for *tripa* imbalance. So we can use Kunye for three of the five elements.

This morning we spoke about *lung, tripa,* and *pekan*: Kunye can be used for *tripa* as well as for *lung*. But of course we use different oils in each case. Why do we use Kunye more commonly to treat *tripa* and *lung*? Because both *tripa* and *lung* have a "light nature." And both also have a "rough" nature. *Lung* dries the body essence because the nature of the wind is rough. *Tripa* dries the body essence because it is heat. The action is different, but the result is similar. Both lighten the body and both make it difficult to sleep, difficult to concentrate, with short temper, anxiety, depression, sorrow, and so forth. So what we need to do is to make the body a little heavier, a little smoother. When we need this kind of treatment, we use Kunye.

As we said earlier, Kunye is based on oils. *Ku* means applying oils, and traditionally we use ghee. There are two kinds of ghee: aged ghee and fresh ghee. Aged ghee does not mean it is frozen or refrigerated for years; it is kept well at room temperature, natural temperature. Also butter comes from cows eating natural grass, so it is natural, totally organic, as they say in America. These two oils are the most common oils used in Kunye. When working on a *tripa* disorder we use fresh ghee because it has a cool nature. For a *lung* disorder we use aged ghee. The nature of any kind of food becomes warmer and lighter when it gets older, when it ages. Ghee is not the only oil we use; we also have others like sesame oil and mustard seed oil. When we use ghee to treat heat nature, as in a *tripa* disorder, we use fresh ghee; but if the season is autumn, if the person is middle-aged, or if they live in a hot, dry climate, we choose fresh ghee mixed with something like essential sandalwood oil. If it is really a serious case and the person is having a real problem with heat, we can also use essential camphor oil. Oils like sandalwood and camphor have a cool nature, so they are suited for further increasing the cool nature. If we do Kunye for someone who cannot sleep, has heavy anxiety, heavy depression, is very light and cannot focus, and so on, we use aged ghee. If it is a serious case we can add nutmeg oil, or cardamom oil, or ginger oil, thus making the oil extra warm.

In general, when the objective is to maintain the body or keep it in what we could call normal balance, we mostly use sesame oil. Especially if the season is winter, if the location is windy, or if the person is older than sixty or so, we generally use normal sesame oil. On the other hand, if we want to maintain the body in health and the person is middle-aged or the season is autumn, we use lavender oil. When we work with Kunye and our main target is a *tripa* problem or a *lung* problem, we use an approach we call *chumigchu sum*: we apply the oil, then rub it in, then later wipe or clean the oil from the body. Why do we need to clean the oil afterwards? You remember that yesterday we discussed a type of *tripa* called complexion-clearing bile that is located on the skin, in the pores. If we block the pores they do not exchange the fresh air, and then contaminated air gets blocked and we will have skin disorders. For this reason we need to clean or open the pores, so we wipe the oils so they do not accumulate or block the path. We can use many different powders to clean or wipe the skin, but the best is chickpea flour because as with all members of the lentil family, it is light, rough, and well suited for absorbing the oil from the body. In addition to absorbing the oil, since the nature of chickpeas is cool, it creates freshness. It is also a treatment for the skin. So if you apply oil treatment for a *tripa* problem it is good to clean afterwards, and using chickpea flour is the best.

For *lung* disorders, if we are using oil treatment it is good to keep the oil on our body at least for twelve hours. This is because for oil applied on the body to be truly effective, it takes a certain amount of time to penetrate into the body. It is just like we would not put on lotion immediately before taking a shower. Keeping the oil on the body a little longer is better because it gives the heaviness, thickness, and smoothness of the oil a chance to work and penetrate into the body.

At this point I would like to introduce my colleague Aldo Oneto. He has been practicing Tibetan Kunye for the last eleven years. Although he does not speak the Tibetan language, he knows about Tibetan medicine. This may also be a good opportunity for you to find out more about the subject, and if you are really interested you can learn and become an instructor. As Doctor Kunchok said yesterday, you can learn and apply this practice and in time you can specialize in this type of traditional medicine.

So Aldo is preparing the oils and will give you a demonstration.

One important thing for Kunye is to have a very comfortable base, like a mattress or some other kind of padding. During a Kunye treatment it is a good idea to put something like pillows or cushions under the feet so the body can rest in a horizontal line. Otherwise the hips tend to drop down and this can be uncomfortable.

As we said, *ku* means to apply oils, so of course the patient needs to take off most clothes. Also when we do Kunye, in addition to the fact that the nature of oil is warm, you can make it even warmer by heating it to get quicker results. The aim of Kunye is to apply the oil well so that it penetrates into the skin and then does its work. Our body is made of skin, muscles, fat, and bones, and between them are a lot of channels. This is the basis of our physical body structure. If the outer body – meaning the muscles and skin – are contracted instead of flexible, the tendons and ligaments, including the neural system become a little tight as well. Until we release that tightness or tension we cannot feel better. If that tightness has existed for a long time, it can cause dysfunctions and over time can even cause serious diseases. This is why oil treatments are very important as a means to release tension. Outer tensions not only make problems deeper; once we have problems in the nervous system or in the joints, that situation can bounce back to the muscles and skin and cause them to become even more tense and tight. If this continues a little longer it can gradually affect the organs as well because the outer and inner body are connected by the channels. And then the effects are not only physical but can slowly also lead to unhappiness and mental problems. This is why the application of oil, accompanied by rubbing and heating, is very important.

When we apply oil we need to follow certain steps. The first is apply the oil. The aim of applying oil is to make the body smooth, calm, and so on. When we apply oil, the problem we are trying to address is not on the skin, but rather is related to the *lung* humor. Where is *lung* located? It is in the channels: the channels are like a road and the *lung* is like a passenger. We can also imagine the *lung* as a vehicle that carries all the fluids, all the energies, where they need to travel, from up to down, or out to in, or in to out, wherever they need to travel. To get to that level it is not enough to simply apply the oil; we also need to rub it in to try to develop the heat. We call that part solar, which means warming up. So the technique is to warm up and try to work the oil in; we apply oil on the skin but it goes a little deeper and works on the muscles, on the fat level, so we try to create heat. In a way our body has qualities like plastic: in warm and smooth periods we can stretch it and it is flexible; in cold, frozen periods it becomes very rigid. In that case we need to first apply oil to make it smooth, then create heat so it becomes flexible again.

The technique Aldo is demonstrating now mainly involves working on the vertebrae. The vertebrae are the central column of the body. If we compare the body to a house, it would be like the central beam of the house. Whether the roof is stable or not and how good the walls are all depend on that beam. So, working on the vertebrae is very important. Vertebrae are like bones, but they are not strong; they are very fragile. A vertebra is a joint consisting of three pieces of bone. Inside it is hollow. Inside the vertebra is the nerve. For this reason when you work on vertebrae you should not press too hard. If we dislocate a vertebra or something happens to it, it can squeeze or pinch the spinal cord and that can cause unexpected results: in the worst case, it can even lead to paralysis. So when we work on a vertebra it is best to work with thumbs rather than with the elbows or heavy objects.

The trapezius muscle is one of the very heavy muscles. It is also one of the largest muscles in the body. It is not a soft, tender muscle, but more a thick, hard muscle. It has a very important responsibility. One is that the muscle is a link between the trunk of the body and the important limbs to the head. It also plays a major role in moving the joints. It is very easy for this muscle to get tired. So massage on that muscle is very important to release all tensions in the shoulders, neck, nape, and also the upper part of our back. When we do Tibetan Kunye, of course we need to use our hands. We use our hands mainly and sometimes we also use our elbows. The point of Tibetan Kunye is not to act on deep tissue. The Tibetan Kunye we now practice at the Shang Shung Institute is not something we made up; it is original. We have divided it into about ten different categories. I am not saying we have created a new kind of Kunye. As we said before, Kunye has thousands years of history in Tibetan medicine. Kunye can be used in two ways: as prevention or as a treatment. What I explained before and what Aldo is showing now is a basic, general, or common Kunye. We can generally call it preventive Kunye. It is what in America they call relaxation massage. But we also have pathological treatments. When choosing a treatment for specific physical problems we decide whether the treatment should be deep or not deep.

The technique Aldo is demonstrating now is meant to stretch the vertebrae. We are habituated to certain body positions, so it is very important when we are sitting that we sit straight, try to have the back straight, because if our body is straight then our veins are straight; if the channels are straight whatever needs to travel through them flows quicker and faster and smoother. If we are sitting straight also the vertebrae are not squeezing one another, they have a little space, so they have a more healthy balance, one is not pushing the other one down. But we tend to ignore our posture, so often we like to sit in a wrong way. What happens is that one vertebra pushes the other so they look like good friends, stacked on top of each other; one has bigger attachment to another, it is like they want to stay together. As a result we have pain in the lower back, this is a very common problem. Also sometimes our body looks a little shrunken. Why? Because our vertebrae are stacking on top of each other. So this technique is meant to stretch vertebrae, to make it easier to create the distance between the vertebrae.

We not only do Kunye massage on the muscles, tendons, and ligaments, we also work on the points. Yesterday Doctor Lhusham Gyal showed the five chakra points and gave a demonstration of power points at the chakras. When we talk about chakras, the term means something like a station or an intersection, a very busy intersection with uninterrupted going and coming, a lot of movement. Chakra means something like that; there are a lot of things coming and a lot of things leaving. There are major chakras, minor chakras, and more subtle chakras. Like an international airport, a local airport, and a bus station: all are busy but on a different level. So since the chakras have a lot of movement, a lot of interaction, it is very easy for the wind to go up or down or get disorganized in some way. We work on the major chakras trying to release the minor chakras. You can imagine when an international airport is backed up for some reason, how many passengers will be stuck there, how many energies will be held up there. With the chakras it is the same. But if everything is moving and people are able to go where they need to go, they waste less energy and are more free. The same happens when we work on the major chakras using heat, as Doctor Kunchok explained. We can use poultices composed of medicinal substances: mostly we use caraway seeds and cardamom seeds. With this kind of herbs we make a poultice and then we heat it and put it on the chakras. Once the chakra is released and functioning, the memory will improve, the circulation, the body movement, everything will improve.

When we do Kunye therapy, after we use a strong technique we follow up with a soft technique to prevent the side effects. If the first technique we used has some side effects, we try to remedy that with a softer technique. Sometimes when we strongly press on an area it could be that we press on a nerve or a vein, it could be that we create a little bruise, something compresses in that area. If we drive a car over a rubber tube it will become flat. If water needs to pass through that tube after we flattened it, the water cannot move. We do not want to leave any tubes flat, so this is why we have a secondary technique to fix anything that may have gone wrong with the first technique. This way we will not have side effects from a Kunye treatment. People often pay hundreds of dollars for some kind of massage treatment and when they come back after a few days they are not able to move. That is why Kunye includes a preventive technique, a method to repair or prevent side effects.

Now if anyone has questions we can answer them while Aldo finishes what he is doing.

Q: A lot of people believe that Ayurveda and Chinese medicine are the same as Tibetan medicine: can you tell us the main differences?

A: Honestly I do not know much about that because I am neither expert in Ayurveda nor in traditional Chinese medicine. So it is a little difficult for me to explain in detail what the differences are. But as Chögyal Namkhai Norbu said the other day, the root of Tibetan medicine comes from Tibet. So when we have a different root we can say that the trunk is different and the branches will be different as well. It is true that these three medicines have a lot in common, but lots of things are also different. For example, when Ayurvedic medicine explains the humors *vata*, *pita*, and *kapha*, each humor is composed by two elements, but in Tibetan medicine when we talk about *lung*, *tripa*, and *pekan*, *lung* and *tripa* are each composed only of one element, what we could call a single duality, while *pekan* is composed of two elements, earth and water, so we could call it a dual duality.

What Aldo is doing now is working on the points. Right now he is working on the first vertebra according to Tibetan medicine, which is the equivalent to the seventh in Western medicine. This point is considered one of the major *lung* points. This point is good for making *lung* calm down.

The next points to treat are the sixth and seventh vertebrae as counted in the Tibetan system. The sixth is the life-sustaining point and the seventh is the physical heart point. All three points are very good for helping patients who have had a heart attack or who have irregular heartbeat, weakness of the heart muscle such as weak circulation, weak memory, for instance not being able to remember what happened the day before, a lot of fear in the heart due to a lack of trust in themselves and a loss of confidence, or depression or anxiety. For all these conditions, the points on the first vertebra as counted according to Tibetan medicine and then the sixth and seventh counting from the first are extremely effective. They are also good for treating sleep problems and short temper. Short temper in itself is not really the problem, but what short temper can cause is fewer friends; fewer friends leads to loneliness, and loneliness then creates depression and so on. So it is a very simple, stupid thing that leads to big problems. To prevent this kind of thing ending up with a need to take anti-depressants or some heavy kind of medicine like that, it is very good to use this type of technique. Believe me, I have used this technique for the last thirty years. I have applied it in remote areas in the high mountains in Tibet and then came to the

United States, a busy country, and the same technique works perfectly here. So take my word for it and then try to apply it yourself.

This kind of Kunye generally is more than just massage. When we have a full understanding of the medical theory behind it, we call it Kunye therapy or Kunye treatment. When we apply this kind of knowledge we can have quick results. And receiving the treatment is also very joyful. It is easy to apply and inexpensive. If someone needs to take anti-depressants you can imagine how much they will spend for the pills. Plus, it is not as if you can take just one pill one day or thirty pills for one month and resolve the problem. Once you start, you need to take the medicine for the rest of your life, and at one point it will not work anymore and so you will need another one. In the meantime there are also a lot of side effects. A treatment like Kunye, on the other hand, is simple, effective, and inexpensive, and there are no side effects. That is the idea Chögyal Namkhai Norbu was talking about the other day: Tibetan culture and Tibetan medicine can benefit all sentient beings.

Thank you for your attention. Thanks also to Aldo for the demonstration.

PRESENTATION

PHUNTSOG WANGMO
Conception and Embryology According to Tibetan Medicine

January 14, morning

Today our subject is embryology; it concerns the baby's development and the mother's care and is a very important topic. If we look at our personality and lifestyle or our character, each person has a different one. Where does this beautiful character come from? Why do we have this kind of character? This very important question goes back to conception, which is the root where our character comes from. Sometimes, because of your character, you may not like other people, sometimes you may not like your own character and wish it was a little different. Character is something that stays with you for the whole life. You can train to make it smoother or change it a bit; in fact one thing that the Buddhist teaching does is also to help one train to change it. I am not saying to change it totally, but to change something, making it more suitable.

The Seven Natural Constitutions
In Tibetan medicine we talk of seven different natural constitutions: three are made up of a single humor; three of two humors combined; and one of a combination of three humors. The three constitutions

characterized by only one humor are: the *lung* constitution, the *tripa* constitution, and the *pekan* constitution. Three constitutions are dual, which means two elements or two humors are present in each nature, such as *lung* and *tripa* united, or *pekan* and *tripa* united, or *pekan* and *lung* united. And the last constitution is the combination of the three humors together, in equal proportion.

Why do we have these seven constitutions? Firstly they derive from the substances of the conception from father and mother, that is to say the sperm and the egg, depending on which element is more predominant. Second they come from the mother's diet, behavior, and life circumstances during the time of pregnancy. Because the baby starts from nothing and in nine months develops to be quite big, during the growth in the mother's womb, diet, behavior, and life circumstances of the mother are very relevant for the child's future character. It is important that they are in balance, so the character of the baby will be balanced as well.

Cause and Period of Conception

As we said yesterday, the mother's egg and father's sperm are based on the five elements; but we also have what is called consciousness. So the father's sperm, the mother's egg, and a consciousness are the fundamental elements to conceive a baby.

Women cannot conceive before they are twelve. From the age of twelve there is such possibility, but until they are fifteen the body is not really ready. For that reason traditionally in Tibet the marriage age starts from fifteen years old. It does not mean that all Tibetan people marry at fifteen, but that according to the tradition it can happen. After the age of fifty it is again difficult to conceive, because menstruation stops. Before twelve there is not enough substance for conception and after fifty again there is not enough substance to conceive. In any case, whether to conceive or not conceive, the function of the body in general is to hold, to maintain life. In Tibetan medicine we call this *zung dun*. *Zung* means sustaining, *dun* means seven. It is to say that the seven constituents of the body maintain or sustain the life. Which are these seven constituents? They are: the essence of food or chyle, blood, muscles, fat, bones, bone marrow, and reproductive fluid. So you see, reproductive fluid is the last, the pure part.

When we eat, food is roughly divided through digestion into pure and impure parts. The pure part goes to the liver and that essence of food transforms into blood. The pure part of blood is again processed and divided into two parts, pure and impure. The pure part goes into the muscles, regenerates them and again divides into pure and impure. The pure transforms into fat. When it gets into the fat it regenerates the fat substances and then divides again into pure and impure. The pure goes to the bones. When it gets into the bones it regenerates the bone substances and then, again digested, is divided into two parts. The pure goes to the bone marrow. When it gets into the bone marrow it regenerates the bone marrow substances and the pure part transforms into the reproductive fluids. This means that to create the reproductive substances, first we need to build well the mechanics of the body substances, including blood, muscles, fat, bones, bone marrow, and so forth. Females under twelve years old are still in childhood. The food they consume is just building the body and not enough substance can go to the reproductive fluids.

For men it is also the same, but the base is a little bit different, because when we talk of men and women, women have a predominance of solar energy and men have a predominance of lunar energy. In women the solar energy develops quicker, but it also decays quicker. In men the development of the lunar energy is a slower process, but it lasts longer. For this reason, as we said, for men is best not to lose the reproductive fluid before eighteen, because the body is still not adequately developed. If you consider the physical aspect, their body may look strong, but inside something is still missing. Once their body is fully developed, their vitality lasts longer, so men over sixty can still have children while female after fifty normally cannot have children anymore.

Physical Obstacles to Conception

During the fertile period, which lasts about thirty-eight years, it does not mean that women can have a child at any time. There are two causes that may hinder conception; one is physical and the other concerns the fluids.

As far as the physical part, for females, but for men also, two organs are most important: the reproductive ones and the kidneys. If one of the two is weak it is difficult to conceive. Four things can happen, affecting either the organs or reproductive fluids: 1) *lung* disorder; 2) *tripa* disorder; 3) *pekan* disorder; and 4) provocation problems.

When there is a *lung* disorder the color of the menstruation or of the sperm is a little darker, less in quantity, and a little rough to the touch. The quantity is insufficient, the quality is too rough, and so it is not able to hold and cannot conceive.

When there is a *tripa* disorder the effects are: again the quantity is less; it becomes a little dry, like a paste, not fluid, the temperature is high, the color is a little dark yellowish. Both the quantity and the quality do not allow for conception because the temperature is too high, when it meets with the egg it boils, it dries the egg, so cannot conceive.

When there is a *pekan* disorder the effects are: excess in quantity, the quality is very heavy, like lubrication, it looks like mucus and sometimes appears like a paste, small balls accompany the liquid. The quantity level is too much; even if the quantity level succeeds to conceive, the quality level does not allow it to stay in place because it is too heavy and too cold.

When there is contamination or provocation, many symptoms can arise and everything is a little unpredictable. Sometimes there are the same symptoms as for *lung* or *tripa*: the quality is dry, thus the reproductive fluids are lacking quantity. Sometimes men lose sperm without any reason. These are some examples of provocations. They have multiple symptoms, and again the capacity of conceive is missing.

All of these four can be treated. Treatment again is based on the five elements, as we described yesterday.

Karmic Obstacles to Conception

If the physical body is suitable for conceiving, another factor can block the conception; this is what we call karma. For having a child, in Tibetan medicine and especially in Buddhism, we think there must be a very strong karmic connection. To be born in a family is not something that you accidentally choose, such as if you are good you selected a good family, and if you are stupid you selected a bad family, it is not like this. Whatever family we have is connected by karma. So, to have a child or not have a child also depends on your karma and merits.

If the father's sperm and the mother's egg are healthy and these two persons are in union, this is the first cause, or the seed, to conceive. Then we need a consciousness. So, the father is ready, the mother is ready, but the baby's consciousness needs to enter into the womb. According to Buddhism and Tibetan medicine life is not something brand new; the baby is new, but that consciousness has been around for many generations, many lifetimes. That is why our main concern is the cause and effect. We say that if you do something bad in this life you have to pay in the next life or at the end of this very life. That is also why fifty years ago, when Tibetans ran Tibetan government, our laws were based on the ten dharmas, or ruled by the Dharma. At that time they were called "the ten actions of society"; among them, three regard the physical level, four the voice, three the mind.

The three regarding the physical body are: killing; stealing; and sexual misconduct.

These actions are prohibited.

The four regarding the voice are: lying; gossiping, or saying bad things about people; harsh speech; and interfering between good friends or between Master and students to make them split, and so on.

The three regarding the mind are: hating or attacking a person; wishing something bad for a person and being happy if something bad happens to them; and wrong view, like for example thinking that if you kill someone you do not have to worry because there is not cause and effect.

We call these "the ten laws of the society." The Dharma kings ruled the nation according to these laws. In the Himalayan mountains there were no police patrolling for twenty-four hours, but somehow we believed that if we did something bad, in this life or in the following ones we would have to pay back: maybe in the next life we would not be born as humans but as animals, we would not even have the capacity to pay back. This is our main worry and it is also something that prevents us from committing negative actions.

Therefore, in order to conceive and have a joyful and beautiful baby you have to have certain merits. Where would these merits come from? As I said before, you try to avoid the ten negative actions and try to perform the ten positive actions. Instead of killing beings or animals you try to save animals' lives. Instead of lying to people you try to be honest and tell the truth. Instead of hating someone or plotting something bad against him, try to cultivate love and kindness. Instead of feeling happy when something bad happens to someone, try to cultivate and develop compassion. If we have good enough compassion, good enough loving kindness, enough saving of other beings' lives that are suffering, that is part of accumulating merits. Whatever you want to do, you need to do it sincerely and not for your own purpose. This is also the essence of the Dharma. Buddha said: "Taking as example your own body do not harm other beings." Sometimes we think: "It is a small ant, it does not matter!" and you kill it. But this ant thinks it is big and beautiful enough to have a life and a family and is not willing to die. This being has attachment to its own body and life. This is also part of the respect for nature and for all sentient beings.

Conception and Embryology

So, if you have good merits, good karma, plus healthy sperm and egg, which are the substances to conceive, and a consciousness that is ready, then conception can occur. The Tibetans explain many ways in which the consciousness enters the mother's womb. It looks like that also depends on where the consciousness is coming from. Some enter through the crown chakra, some through the ring finger to the heart chakra, or more commonly they enter through the breathing canal, that is to say through the breath.

When the consciousness enters the mother's womb it has a sort of feeling. Searching for its parents is like arriving in a large, crowded station, looking for someone to pick you up; sometimes it takes a very long time. When it is time to enter, the consciousness has the sensation that it is rainy, windy, and there are a lot of people running and trying to find a shelter, a safe place they can enter. There are very few consciousnesses that know where they are going. When common consciousnesses enter into the mother's womb, they have no idea of where they are going; they know they are looking for a safe place and that they are entering a shelter where they can feel quiet, warm, protected, and safe. They feel happy there. From the moment they enter the womb until they come out, thirty-eight weeks pass.

The first week after the father's sperm, the mother's egg, and the consciousness have met, the substance is like milk mixed with yogurt, very liquid. In the second week, the milk assumes an egg's shape, a little oblong. In the third week it becomes as solid as yogurt.

In the fourth week, the fetus develops and establishes its gender. If someone prefers to have either a boy or a girl that would be the time to do related practices. Once the fourth week has passed, the gender is already formed. In the fifth week the umbilical cord is formed. In the sixth week, our central and side channels form from the base of the umbilical cord. The upper part of the central channel goes up to the crown chakra and the lower goes down to the secret chakra. The two side channels, called *roma* and *kyangma,* go to the nose and end in the nostrils.

When the seventh week comes, the eyes appear, symbolic eyes. In the eighth week, based on the symbolic eyes, the head forms.

In the ninth week the upper and lower part of the body can be distinguished, so the trunk of the body, the shape of the body is formed.

When the tenth week comes, the shoulders and hips are formed. This starts from the third month. At that time the shoulders are still not protruding, they are just appearing. This is called the period or the stage of the fish. At that time the mother can easily lose the baby through miscarriage or some secondary causes. Until that point the mother feels morning sickness, like nausea and these kinds of things. As we said before, in the fourth week, when the gender appears in the fetus, the mother feels tired, emotionally either happy or unhappy, and also feels that her breasts are swelling. She has desire to eat foods with many different tastes. Depending on whether the fetus is going to be a boy or a girl, the mother will have two different desires. If the fetus is going to be a boy she would like to eat more spicy and sour, if is going to be a girl she will like more sweet things. She will be attracted to eating, drinking, wearing ornaments, and so forth. So we say this is not a desire of the mother, but of the fetus. At that time you need to try to satisfy the mother, otherwise the fetus will feel unsatisfied. So, traditionally, whatever the mother wants we try to give it to her.

Then, starting from the eleventh week, the shoulders and hips are more prominent. Not only the shoulders, but also the sense organs are more evident.

When the twelfth week comes, the upper arms and upper legs and the five solid organs appear.

When the thirteenth week comes, the six hollow organs appear.

When the fourteenth week comes, which is in the fourth month, arms and legs appear.

When the fifteenth week comes, the lower part of arms and legs is more established.

When the sixteenth week comes, the twenty digits appear, meaning the ten fingers and the ten toes.

When the seventeenth week comes, the channels are linked throughout the body. Remember that, starting from the sixth week, we have the central channel and the two side channels; the network of secondary channels in the upper and lower and inner and outer body is linked through these three channels.

When the eighteenth week comes, muscles and fat develop.

When the nineteenth week comes, ligaments and tendons develop. Ligaments link bones to bones, tendons connect muscles to muscles. So now the body is not only connected through the channels but also the upper and lower parts of the body are connected as well.

When the twentieth week comes, all the bones are formed. Certain bones also contain bone marrow.

When the twenty-first week comes, the fetus is covered by skin. At this time basically the whole body is formed. We call this moment the period or stage of the turtle. It means that now the baby has shoulders and legs completely formed. It is also growing up so it is pushing the mother's abdomen, we can see something protruding. Some women have a big belly while others not so much. In Tibetan medicine we say that if the fetus is a boy he is emotionally attached to females and against male, so he is facing towards the mother and the mother's bottom part of the belly is protruded. If the fetus is a girl, emotionally she is more attached to men. So she faces towards the father and against the mother, pushing back, therefore the belly sides are directed outwards. If you look at the backside of the mother the sacrum is more protruded and the front not so very much. If they are twins the sides of the mother's belly are more protruded because the babies inside are settled face to face, so the two sides of the mother are more protruded and her belly looks kind of empty in the front.

Starting from the sixth month, in the twenty-second week, the sense organs become bigger and more visible.

In the twenty-third week, nails and hair appear. Nails and hair are the impure parts of the bones; this means that now the baby's bones are well formed.

In the twenty-fourth week, the five solid organs and the six hollow organs become clear and visible. At that time the fetus experiences happiness or unhappiness, and starts to have the feeling of conscious-ness. Either it likes or does not like hot or cold. At that moment, when the fetus is showing emotions, the mother also feels more emotional. During all this period, which lasts about two or three weeks, the mother goes through an emotional transition. So, the mother experiences strong emotions in the fourth week and then again in the twenty-fourth week, when the baby is having emotional understanding.

When the twenty-fifth week comes, the baby is starting to inhale, so the air element is circulating into the baby's body. This means that now the baby is capable to develop by himself, because the wind is circulating, which means that everything is circulating.

When the twenty-sixth week comes, the fetus has a clear memory and for the first time starts to remember things. At that moment the awareness of the present is vague, the awareness of the future is vague; mainly the fetus has memories of the past, of its previous life. For this reason, at the moment of birth some babies are laughing, some are crying, and some look very scared, like they are having a nightmare. We believe that this kind of energy comes from the past, because birth is very close to past life, so it remembers and shows sort of symptoms.

Starting from the twenty-seventh till the thirty-first week everything becomes bigger, more clear and visible.

From thirty-first to the thirty-sixth week everything develops. At that time, if you have a premature birth the baby can survive because everything is already formed. Starting from the thirty-first week to the thirty-fifth, one day the mother is stronger and another day the fetus can be stronger, so the mother's physical strength comes and goes. When the mother is strong, with a good complexion and clear voice, the fetus is a little weak. When the mother is weak and tired, the fetus is stronger. Sometimes in that period there can be a premature birth. If the baby is born when the mother is in the strong phase, it is very difficult for him to survive, because on that day his energy is weak. If you have a premature birth when the mother is having a weak day, the baby will survive because his energy is strong.

Once we get to the thirty-sixth week, the fetus inside the mother womb is starting to have feelings of dislike to stay there. It feels a little bit sad there; it feels the space is small, stinky, sticky, cold, and wet, not a nice place to be.

When the thirty-seventh week comes, the baby starts to search for the gate. If you have the help of a midwife, in Tibetan medicine, between the thirty-sixth and the thirty-seventh week we check how the baby's head is turning. Especially in the thirty-seventh week, we help the mother turn the head of the baby down close to the gate, because sometimes, if the mother is weak, the turning of the baby is not that fast. If the baby is weak he tries to search the gate, he goes a little further but cannot continue because he is weak and sometimes remains in a diagonal position. For this reason we try to help the baby turn in a healthy manner.

So, for the period of nine months and ten days we speak of embryology; the fetus is developing in the mother's womb. We basically divide the nine months into three parts. For the first three months the baby is still liquid, soft, and this is the stage of the fish, when the fetus can easily be lost. What can we do in order to keep the baby inside healthy and also to keep the mother happy? We can apply three things: diet, behavior, and therapies.

Maintaining Health of Mother and Child During Pregnancy

As far as the diet, in the first three months of pregnancy it is very important to try to keep the wind low. Why? Because one of the functions of wind is to open or close the gate, so we do not want to open the gate unnecessarily, at the wrong time, and lose the baby. Therefore it is good to eat something nutritious but with warm nature. Nutritious food helps calm the wind down, while food with a warm nature is appropriate because we want to plant the seed. We describe the father's sperm as the seed and the mother's egg as the field, and when we plant a seed, the field needs heat, a warm temperature, otherwise nothing will grow.

Which other kind of food is good? Dairy products are good, meat products are good, and fish and chicken would be the best at that moment because fish has warm nature. Pork, on the other hand, is cold and heavy.

In the following three months the child is growing in the abdomen and needs to build his body. The mother's mouth is feeding two bodies, so again, nutritious food is important. In this period heat is not as important as before because the seed is already planted and growing, therefore keeping a neutral temperature is enough. But in order to grow it still needs soil and water. So nutritious food, like dairy products, meat products, and grain products, is still good. In this period lentils and buckwheat are not good since these two groups do not have the capacity to build things, as they have a cold and rough nature. Rough is good to clean the fat but not to build the fat.

In the last three months the body is already built, so the job is to maintain it. Again the mother needs nutritious but warm nature food that is more neutral. Neutral is good for maintaining. If the mother eats too many heavy things, the baby will grow too large, then there will be another problem. In this period it is good to eat small quantities of buckwheat. I am not saying that now you can have only lentils and buckwheat, but mixed food. It is good to eat sweet things combined with some bitter tastes like lentils.

Throughout the pregnancy, oil treatment and some warm compresses are very important for the mother, because the nature of oil is heavy, sticky, and smooth. The nature of wind is light, rough, mobile, so oil treatment helps to keep the wind down. Keeping the wind low in the first three months helps keep the baby inside; in the second three months it helps the baby grow healthy; in the last three months it helps the baby's balance, and in the last hours it helps open the gate so we can have a good labor. If during the pregnancy we are able to keep the wind calm, after giving birth the woman will not be strongly affected emotionally. One of the big issues for a woman after the birth are emotional problems, so this is prevented. In Tibetan medicine this is how to conceive and how to develop.

Postpartum Care

When we arrive at the birth itself, the first thing is to observe the auspicious or inauspicious signs, a sort of welcoming the baby in the family or in the society. If the baby is faced up, has no teeth, the umbilical cord is wrapped on the upper back, and the baby comes out crying with a strong voice, we call these positive signs. Positive or negative does not mean good or bad for the family, they are good or bad for the baby's health or for his life. We consider it less positive if the face is down and the baby comes with teeth. But positive or less positive is not the main point; the important thing is having a healthy baby.

Once the baby is born we wash him in water and milk; this symbolizes for the baby having nutrition and the white path. Washing him in rough water may not feel good to him. Water and milk is like lubrication, like jelly, is sticky and soft and the direct contact of our hands is also very rough for the baby, that is why we add milk, like a cream for the body. In Tibetan medicine a lot of positive symbolism is connected with milk, for instance, it signifies a journey on the white path, into the land of nutrition, and so on.

After birth, caring for the mother is important, both trying to keep the wind down and preventing her from infections. Why do we need to keep the wind down? Labor is a big job, plus there is a loss of blood, so wind can become unbalanced. And why do we need to pay attention to infections? Because during labor there may be damage to the womb or the cervix. Sometimes also some pieces of placenta or of other material can remain in the uterus and this can cause her difficulties in later conceptions, or infections due to uterine problems. For that reason it is very important in the first week to take some herbs for the inflammation to make sure that there are no complications.

In the first six months the baby basically lives on the mother's milk, on breast-feeding. Again for the mother it is important to eat good, nutritious food with a warm nature. Then, starting from the sixth month, we can start to introduce food. In Tibetan medicine the development of the baby is very important. As we said before, we have earth, air, fire, water, and space elements, to build these elements we need the content of food. In Tibet we do not have vitamin pills, so we have to introduce these substances with food. Bones are the main structure of the body, are like the base, the foundations, very important, so what we do is consume bone broth. Bones have the highest calcium content, so to build the bones we need calcium and vitamin D. In Tibet we do not have that, so we drink bone broth, milk, and dairy products. In order to build the iron substances we eat different green vegetables including spinach and lentils. In order to build the muscles, meat itself is good, so we introduce all of these things in the diet.

Thank you for listening.

PRESENTATION

KUNCHOK GYALTSEN
*Diet Based on Personal, Seasonal,
and Environmental Conditions*

January 14, afternoon

Tonight I would like to talk to you briefly about food and drink in Tibetan medicine. It is a big topic, impossible to cover everything in one hour; therefore I will briefly discuss the principles of food and drink and the practical application of these principles. This talk is also meant for people who are not going to become doctors, otherwise it would go more in depth and would be more complex.

Part One: The Nature of the Human Body
As we know, we all have a physical body with its vital and hollow organs. Food and drink mainly pass through the hollow organs and finally go to all parts of the body. Why do we drink and eat every day? Our body is made of the five elements: earth, water, fire, wind, and space. The elements also form the universe; so every day we take part of the universe into our body in order to maintain it for a certain time.

Of course, we enjoy food and drink but the purpose of consuming it is to maintain our life and our physical body. That is why in Buddhist philosophy we say that each time we eat and drink we should not think we are doing it for the body to become bigger or stronger or whatever we wish; the only reason for doing it is to keep our body healthy, so that we can do a lot of meaningful things. As you can imagine, if we did not have a healthy body our life would be meaningless. Therefore food is very important. Everybody eats every day, so we need to understand a little about the concept of digestion in Tibetan medicine.

Our body is formed by the five elements, which are different from the five elements in traditional Chinese medicine. Here they are real material elements. In Tibetan we call them *zug*, which are the materials that make up our body. The elements are earth, water, fire, and wind, plus the space element. In Tibetan terms these five elements are related to *lung, tripa*, and *pekan*.

The Three Humors

Many people like to talk about the five elements because they are very commonly described in traditional medicine. However, there are various levels of understanding the five elements. Tibetan medicine looks at the actual material in the physical body. Here on this diagram you can see a circle or sphere, like a cell, and in terms of Western medicine, our body is like one big mass of cells. Our body contains millions of small cells; in Tibetan terminology they are called *dul trarab*. So the smallest subdivision of the body is the cell.

Each part of the body has three functions called *lung, tripa*, and *pekan* in Tibetan. If you want to understand a little about Tibetan medicine you must understand these terms. This concept is just common sense. At a macro level *pekan* is a water-earth combination. We can touch our body: without *pekan* we do not have a body. We have this physical body because of the combination of earth and water. Our physical body also has heat inside it. The degrees of heat are different, but there is heat in it. Because of heat, earth and water are always alive. In order to be alive or change, there is wind or gas, which moves things. Wind or gas pushes *tripa* to interact with the combination of earth and water, and that is how we are alive.

In Western medicine or Western science there are many substances in food that we need in our bodies, like vitamins, and so on. Similarly, Tibetan medicine has the concept that it is from food that we take parts of *pekan*, *tripa*, and *lung* into our body every day. It is like a car: you need to put gasoline in it every day otherwise it will not move. This is a similar idea; that is why we eat food every day.

Body Functions

According to the first part of the *Gyüzhi*, the *Four Tantras*, *lung*, *tripa*, and *pekan* each has five subcategories or functions. These fifteen categories can actually make complete sense of how the body functions.

As we are going to talk about food and drink, we need to concentrate on the stomach. In the stomach, three things work together like teamwork. The first is called *menyam* in Tibetan; it is translated as the fire-accompanying wind; it is *lung* with the function of moving, but there is also heat. In *tripa* there is *tripa juged*; it is like a digestive *tripa*, which is actually heat itself. The third one is *pekan nyaged*, meaning mixing. You must know these three functions. If you want to understand a little about how food is digested you must consider these three.

To simplify, when we eat, food goes into the stomach – you can see in the diagram – and there it becomes chyle. Then we need something to mix the food because our teeth cannot mix it precisely; sometimes we swallow bigger pieces, sometimes smaller.

Another function we need is to heat the food. During this stage, there is a wind that moves in the stomach. It performs a function, like cooking a soup. It is like digestion. The stomach is like a factory where these three bodies are working together: mixing and heating to produce something like cooked food. At the same time they also divide the food. The nutrition part is always sent from the stomach to the liver. The waste is first sent to the small intestine, then to the big intestine, and finally becomes feces. The nutrition is sent to the liver, then to the flesh, then to the fat, then to the bones, and finally becomes reproductive fluids:

the entire process takes seven days. Any kind of nutrition you eat takes one week to reach the final stage.

At this point you can understand that the stomach is very important. If you understand the digestive process, the understanding of food is less important. What kind of food we eat is of course important, but the stomach is more important. If we do not have a good stomach, no matter what we eat, it is useless, because sometimes it is not digested and all goes to waste. Sometimes the waste goes to the liver and the blood becomes contaminated. Today we see a lot of people with bladder-related diseases because they have a bad stomach, plus they eat bad food.

Keeping the stomach warm is very important, but usually we destroy the fire or the heat in the stomach. For example, in the USA if you go to a restaurant you will see many people drinking water with ice. Restaurants always automatically serve water with ice; if they do not do it people will be upset. Then they automatically drink it. Your stomach is empty when you go to a restaurant: if you pour iced water in an empty stomach it becomes very cold. Then you eat steak or fish, i.e. oily food, and the food just stacks up. Many people get fat because a lot of fatty waste is transferred to the liver and in the liver some part of the nutrition becomes blood, some part goes to the flesh and then there is a lot of waste flesh, waste fat. That is why people look big and fat, but they are very weak because they do not have much energy.

Another thing people need to understand is that – I do not know about this country; America is more familiar to me – in America, a lot of people take substances like vitamins, vegetable vitamins, a lot of pills, in order to have a stronger body and then they eat very little. They do not take any real food and then their stomach, small intestine, and big intestine shrink because not much stuff goes through. That is also very bad.

Let me give you an example. If you go on vacation and leave your house for one or two months, when you come back the water pipe is dark, rusted. This is similar, because your body needs those normal things to happen; you must make your body normal. I am not saying that taking vitamins is bad; I am just saying that, as a natural person, first we need to act in a natural way. If you have a problem in your body, *then* you can take vitamins or supplements because they can save your life. So, they are also important. Naturally we have all those functions, so we should use them in a smart way, otherwise we would be going against our natural body. That would be very bad because – if you in the West believe in Christ – our body is a gift of God or – according to Buddhist philosophy – it is the result of cause and effect. So we must follow our natural way first.

Part Two: Dietary Principles and Application

Principles and Functions of Food

Now we will talk about food. There are thousands of kinds of food, so it is impossible also for me to know them all, but using the theory of Tibetan medicine we can understand almost all foods. Tibetan medicine scholars use their natural taste – that is, their tongue – to classify all food into six categories of tastes. When we eat or drink any kind of food, during the digestion stage in the stomach, the tastes can be summarized into three kinds: sweet, bitter, and sour. These three post-digestion tastes are not very important for you to understand, the important ones are the six categories of tastes. I will explain them one by one.

As regards sweet: there is standard sweet in Tibetan medicine, I will just show you some images since they may help to illustrate. The definition of sweet is "having a pleasant flavor and causing the desire to taste again and again." Maybe this is a bad translation; in Tibetan language it is beautifully described. Sometimes translation frustrates me. I wish you could all understand Tibetan so I could explain the precise meaning. As examples of sweet taste we have sugar, honey, and sweet potatoes; these are the typical sweet flavors.

The definition given for sour is "having the taste produced chiefly by acid, tasting sharp, tart, or tangy." Examples are lemon or lime juice and vinegar. Maybe today we also have passion fruit.

The salty taste is easy for you because you live next to the ocean. The definition is "having a sharp taste at first and then producing saliva in the mouth," such as salt and seaweeds.

The bitter taste is like astringent, the examples are asparagus and coffee, I cannot think of a good plant in the West. Bitter has a very difficult taste; the definition is "having a sharp, biting, unpleasant taste that changes the smell of the mouth after tasting."

The pungent taste is actually like chili, very hot. The definition is "sharply affecting the sense of taste making the tongue and mouth feel a burning sensation," such as garlic and black pepper.

The astringent taste is defined as "a combination of sweet and bitter at first taste, and then the tongue and mouth feel dry and course or rough when the tongue touches the upper hard palate," such as unripe banana or green tea.

The Arithmetic of Taste Combinations

When we talk about these six tastes it sounds like something very common and ordinary, but if you think deeper they are very important because we are eating and drinking every day following the tastes. We must understand that the six categories of tastes we are talking about are the root tastes. Among the six tastes it is very hard to find the purely sweet or purely sour. Among different foods we can probably find sweet, sour, salty, and maybe pungent, others are very difficult to identify because all types of food are a combination of tastes. For example, there can be a double, triple, quadruple, quintuple, or sextuple taste. Examples of double tastes are sweet plus sour, sour plus salty, salty plus pungent, pungent plus astringent. There are six sixes, that makes thirty-six; similarly, thirty-six times six makes two hundred and sixteen. In all there are thousands of tastes. It is quite complex. We, as humans, need to find out about taste.

The Relationship between the Five Cosmo-Physical Elements and the Six Tastes

Why are there so many tastes? It is because they are produced by the earth and the other elements of the natural environment. For example, the sweet taste is mostly produced by the combination of earth and water. Fertilized land produces many sweet kinds of fruit and vegetables because when earth and water are the stronger elements they produce more sweet taste. Similarly, if earth and fire are stronger they produce sour tastes. You can see the similar conditions in this table [water + fire = salty; water + air = bitter; fire + air = pungent; earth + air = astringent]. It is good to understand the six tastes and how you can apply them to your physical situation.

We use our physical body, one of the five senses, to perceive taste. We use our tongue to taste food, but then because different kinds of food are produced by the five elements their functions are also different. In Tibetan medicine we call these functions *nupa gyed*, the eight powers. These powers are: heavy, oily, cool, blunt, light, coarse, hot, and sharp. These are the functions. For example, if you eat a mango your stomach warms up because mango has the power of heat; if you eat a lot of watermelon it reduces the fire in your stomach because it has a cold nature. These are the functions we can understand from the food. You can actually find these potencies in any food, so we can understand the properties of food in this way. And we can also understand medicinal herbs in this way. That is why, in Tibetan herbal medicine, we use these principles to identify the nature of herbs and how to use them.

Table of Potencies Corresponding to Disorders

Furthermore, there are seventeen potencies. The seventeen potencies are how the powers correspond to each other. For example, heavy food is stable. We also use this kind of principle in healing treatments, but this is not too important for you. For example, the nature of a *lung* disorder is coarse, light, cold, subtle, firm, and mobile, so what kind of potencies of food are needed? We need smooth, heavy, warm, stable food. [The nature of a *tripa* disorder is oily, sharp, hot, light, malodorous, and purgative. So we need pale, blunt, cool, heavy, fluid, and dry food. The nature of a *pekan* disorder is oily, cool, heavy, blunt, stable, and smooth. So we need food that is pale, hot, light, sharp, mobile, and coarse]. These things are very technical, so you do not need to worry about them. Now I want to make it simpler for you to understand, so maybe you can use some concepts.

Firstly, you must take care of your stomach. The heat of the stomach is very delicate; so do not drink cold beverages in the morning. When you get up, if you can, before breakfast drink a cup of boiled water. It will heat up your stomach – which is empty in the morning – so that the natural heat in the stomach is strengthened. Moreover, during the night you consume a lot of the water of your body, therefore your stomach sometimes dries up, so adding some water is good.

Never drink heated water; only drink boiled water. If you boil a cup of water until it is reduced by a third, the two thirds remaining will be very good quality water, very good for your stomach. Sometimes the quality of water is good, sometimes it is bad, but generally if you use it boiled even tap water is good. The quality of water also requires careful study. Today people drink bottled water and pay a lot of money for very bad water. Bottled water is especially bad for people with very poor digestive systems. Even the well-known brands and expensive types of water are very bad. Why? Because the water stays in the bottles for many days, it is dead water. In Tibetan medicine the good quality water is spring water, coming from high mountains, water that jumps over the stones and gets sunlight and wind blowing: this kind of water is the best. The worst water is forest water, which come from under the trees and does not see much light and is also stagnant. Bottled water is similar to that. One thing you need to be careful of: the water you boiled today you should drink today; tomorrow you should boil fresh water. You should not keep it over night; it is not good. If you like to drink cold water you can boil it and then cool it in the refrigerator, then it is very good.

Dietary Restrictions

We also make a distinction between accustomed food and non-accustomed food. The best food for good health is the food from where you have grown up. Any kind of food you habitually eat before you are fourteen is your native food. For example, if someone is far away [from his home country] and feels ill, if he can get his native food, meaning the kind of food he was eating until he was about twelve, his body will accept it very well. Particularly old people must eat accustomed food, the food they were eating when they were young. That is very good for their health.

Then there is non-accustomed food. For example, Tibetans eat a lot of meat and dairy products; then if they move to China and eat vegetables every day they get sick. When I was studying in Peking I myself was hospitalized for one month because of that. Therefore always try to keep to your native food. I do not know how people eat here, but in Los Angeles they eat like this: in the morning Indian restaurant; at lunch Japanese restaurant; at night French restaurant; the morning after Mongolian restaurant, then Italian, and then Ethiopian. They eat like this every day. If you grew up this way, fine; but I think it is very difficult.

Then there are bad combinations of food. I am not going to explain it in much detail because the food it includes is not very applicable here. However, there is one thing you must know: today there are very famous chefs, who want to make you eat different kinds of tasty food. They serve various kinds of food combinations, and that is actually a little bit dangerous. For example, if you traditionally have some food combination in this island, it is good, because your ancestors experienced it many times and established the system; but if you make new combinations maybe that is risky. This is only for your information.

The Correct Amount of Food

Another thing that is maybe useful for you to know about is the quantity of food you should eat at every meal. In Tibetan medicine we say you need to divide your stomach into four parts: you fill two parts with solid food, one part with liquid and you leave one part empty. Actually we do not usually have any consciousness of the quantity of food we should eat; we just follow the restaurant business people. Some restaurants serve a big quantity of food, while the so-called fancy restaurants serve very little. Then how can we make a judgment? If we go to a cheap restaurant we eat a lot; if we go to a fancy one we eat very little and when we get home we need to eat more.

We need to understand how much we should eat. How can we measure it? Four [handfuls] is the right quantity to consume. For example, my hand is this big, so I take in four times this much food and drink. We leave one part of the stomach empty; otherwise we cannot digest. This is very helpful, especially if you go to a self-service restaurant. Sometimes people eat a lot there; particularly if they are very hungry they take and eat a lot of food. We are used to having three meals a day. If you want to be healthy you should eat this much at every meal. Because we have different body-sizes, the stomach is different too, and so, our hands can measure precisely how big our stomach is. Then, if you go to a fancy restaurant and they give you too little, it is all right for you to eat more. If you are a mother you have to look at everybody's hands to see how big or small they are and then you serve the food accordingly; do not serve the same amount to everybody. This concept is actually very scientific; in Tibetan medicine we always recommend it. It is really useful, therefore I am happy to share it with you.

Seasonal Dietary Principles

This table is about the seasons. On this island the four seasons are not so clear, so maybe it is not very applicable here, but where there are normally four seasons we can apply in this way. For example we consider March-April to be early spring [and November-December upper winter]. Maybe, if we take into consideration four seasons – spring, summer, fall, and winter – instead of six it will be easier.

In the precise [lunar] calendar, the dates are different every year, but generally spring includes February, March, and April: the three months when days become longer and nights shorter. During this time you need food with more bitter, pungent, and astringent taste, these are the three tastes that are good for you in springtime.

May, June, and July are considered to be summer and you should take more sweet, sour, and salty tasting food.

August, September, and October are considered to be fall, when sweet, bitter, and astringent tasting food is good.

November, December, and January is winter: sweet, sour, and salty tasting food is good in this period.

Because of the earth turning around the sun, the seasons change and our body changes, too. Let me give some examples. In summer people are very thirsty so they drink a lot. Automatically they think that in summer they need to drink a lot of water – particularly iced, cold water – but actually in summer you need to be very careful about taking very cold drinks because inside our body would be very cold and outside is hot. In winter people automatically eat a lot because inside is warm and we can consume a lot of food and outside is cold.

Individual Characteristics and Food

Now I would like to talk about one's personal nature. This is another vast subject, but I will try to be brief. Although we can divide people into seven categories, it would be a little complicated to cover here, so we can concentrate on three main ones: *lung* nature, *tripa* nature, and *pekan* nature. Here *lung*, *tripa*, and *pekan* are not diseases or problems; they are just our natural, unaltered features. All of us have these characteristics in our body.

The characteristics of people with *lung* nature are: their body size is shorter and thinner, they have dark skin; they are very active, athletic, and talkative. When they walk they are always playing or moving around; they are good at singing and dancing. Maybe at the time Tibetan medical scholars made these studies they based them on Tibetan appearances and behavior and were not aware of Caucasian or Hispanic or Mediterranean people; but in any case this is still applicable. Anyway you can think about it.

Lung nature people naturally like sweet, sour, hot, and bitter food and need to consume these more in order to maintain their health.

The characteristics of people with *tripa* nature are: their body size is medium; their skin is more yellow; they are always sweating, they have a sharp mind; their thinking is very quick; and they are always confident; they are usually thirsty and easily hungry; they like to consume sweet, bitter and astringent food, which therefore are better for them.

People with a *pekan* natural constitution have the following characteristics: their body size is relatively big; they tend to be fat; they have light skin; their body is always cool; they do not like exercise very much; they always tend to sit in one place and they easily feel sleepy; usually their hands too tend to be fat; they are always patient and do not easily get angry; they like to eat pungent, sour, astringent and coarse food which are, therefore, good for them.

Here in the West we often have a problem of obesity. People who are obese like to eat a lot of sweet food and that is a problem because sweet food is not easy to digest. Therefore it is very important that they consume lighter food. What kind of taste is more frequently used or consumed overall among human beings? Usually sweet food is more consumed, in any kind of society. That is why society today has more obesity problems. We need to be careful about how much sweet food we consume. We also know that big people are *pekan*-nature people. We said before that *pekan* is a combination of earth and water, elements that are generally cold; many *pekan*-nature people have a cool body and so their digestive system is slower. Therefore they cannot eat a lot of sweet and oily food. Sour, coarse, hot, and bitter foods are good for them because they are lighter, easier to digest, and leave fewer problems in the body.

Tonight we talked about how the stomach works, the functions of the nature of the body, and how we can apply the six tastes of food and drink based on Tibetan medicine. If you like you can apply these kinds of concepts. Actually I gave you very basic information; I hope this will be useful for you.

We have a few more minutes, if you have any questions, I can answer them.

Q: What quantity of meat is advisable to eat per week?

A: If you grew up with meat you need to eat more meat, while if you grew up as a vegetarian, you do not need to eat very much; but also the quality of meat is important. Today we have artificially fed cows; the quality of their meat is very poor, therefore it is not good to eat too much of it.

I want to emphasize one thing: always try to eat combinations of different kinds of food; do not always eat only vegetables. Vegetables are good, but not if you eat only them. And also do not eat only meat; a combination is good. For example, it is good to eat meat twice or three times a week. People who grew up in Tibet were accustomed to eating a lot of meat. From our experience we found that if they suddenly stopped eating meat it was very difficult for the body to adjust, particularly as they got older. Then a lot of symptoms showed up. Therefore a certain amount of meat is necessary.

You need to be careful about what kind of meat you eat. You need to pay attention to the fatty part of the meat too. In USA people do not like fat, but you need to eat a little bit, not too much. Also here you have to balance. People always go to extremes: if they eat meat they always eat meat. In some diets for losing weight you eat meat every day, no vegetables or other things. They are meat eaters. Vegetarians never eat any meat. These extremes are actually harmful to our system. Combinations are good.

Q: Which attitude should we have while eating? For example, maybe we are eating very good, ecological food but in a stressed way:

is it better to eat whatever but in a relaxed way and thinking about what we are eating?

A: Food is very important for anybody because without it we cannot live long, unless you practice Buddhist *chüdlen*. As normal people we must eat food therefore we have to have the right attitude towards it. I have already mentioned that you should not eat food because you want to look better than anybody else, or for whatever other reason based on the three poisons: attachment, anger, and ignorance. When you eat you need to be comfortable, to have no worries, because if we have enough food on our table we are very lucky. From the Christian point of view this is a gift of God and you are very lucky. From the Buddhist point of view you are very fortunate because you worked hard and then you have some food. So now you enjoy whatever food you have. Maybe in the West or other cultures people always select food, but in Tibet no one would ask: "What would you like to eat?" This question does not exist in Tibet. So, for Tibetan monks and nuns coming to the West the most difficult question to answer is this one. The reason is that we never choose food, we eat whatever is available, because it is our karma to have that food, and so we should appreciate it. Then we eat and enjoy it, and that keeps us stronger.

If you have the wrong attitude you think: "Oh, I shouldn't eat that food! Oh, it's very dirty! Oh, it looks bad!" and then if you eat it, it will definitely make you sick. In the old days times there was no mass-produced food, so one was limited to local produce. Locally produced food also has a hierarchy: some types of food are very much appreciated, others less so. But if you go to a family as a guest, the family will serve you the best food they have. Tibetan Buddhist monks and nuns do not choose to be vegetarian, because lay people offer them whatever food they have, and they eat whatever they receive. This is still the tradition; that is why it is very difficult for us when someone asks, "What would you like to eat?" How do you answer to that?

Attitude is very important; you have asked a good question.

Western science and Western biomedicine have developed new dietary concepts to explain various nutritional concepts. These exist everywhere: not only in the West, but also in the East everybody understands these concepts.

We have now introduced the Tibetan medicine concept: it is very hard to apply within your belief, but if you understand these concepts a little bit and practice them in your daily nutrition I think they will be very beneficial. This is what I wanted to share with you tonight, thank you very much. I wish you all the best.

PRESENTATION

Phuntsog Wangmo
Birth and Pediatrics in Tibetan Medicine

January 15, morning

Today the topic is pediatrics. Childhood diseases and childcare are dealt with in Tibetan medicine in three main sections. The first is called *chipa nyewar chopa* (early child care). It is a sort of continuation from yesterday; it gives advice on childcare from birth till one year of age. The second chapter is about treating diseases; the third is about treating provocations. In the section on provocations, when we refer to pathology, we have five chapters based on provocation diseases in general and one chapter specific for children. In fact, for several reasons, they are easily attacked by provocations during childhood. One reason is because children are very beautiful and cute. A second reason is because they are very innocent, sort of very naive and do not know exactly what they have to do. That is why they can easily be attacked and sort of manipulated. Also in general social care, we pay extra attention to the safety of children, more than for adults, right? Children cannot be left alone, they have to be with an adult, they cannot stay in certain places, they cannot see certain things, and so on. There are a lot of rules for children in the society.

Part One: Pediatrics

Auspicious Signs at Birth

In the first chapter, when we speak of *nyecho*, early childcare, the first thing is to observe the positive or negative signs when the baby is coming out of the mother's womb.

As I said yesterday, if the head is coming first, that is what we call a common birth. If the feet come first, that is an uncommon birth. If the hands come first it is very dangerous. These are the three ways of being born. We also observe if the umbilical cord is wrapped on the upper back, if the central part of the head is a little protruded, a little long, if the forehead is clear, if the hairline is high and the ears are standing straight, not sort of collapsing, if the baby is sucking the mother's milk very strongly; also, if babies are shivering or crying very loudly when they are born, or if they come out face up and their skin is clear, all these are good signs.

Sucking the milk strongly and crying very loudly means that the baby is healthy. This means also that the mucus is not blocking. Because in the mother's womb the baby is basically in liquid, very often the mucus sticks in the throat. Western hospitals have special equipment that sucks the mucus from the baby's mouth and nose. We have it in Tibetan medicine or tradition as well. So if the baby does not cry loudly or there is some blockage, we suck the liquid from his throat. Clear skin means that the baby is totally mature and was born right on time, so it is not a premature birth. A high hairline and a very clear forehead show the future of the baby. Today we do not pay much attention, but traditionally, in order to foresee people's future, the reading of the hairline is very important. The hairline is considered the line of life: if it is large and straight the person has a smooth and passive life. If it is narrow that indicates he will have a somewhat complicated life. Especially in the tradition of India, when a child is born they invite a person to read the baby's body and, based on that, they give him a name. Probably that person is not an ordinary person, but somehow has special qualities. Maybe we also had this kind of thing in ancient Tibet, but today we do not have a special person reading the baby's body and then giving him a name.

Anyway, as soon as the baby is born, the mother needs to pronounce certain auspicious words to the child. As I said yesterday, there is a very strong karmic connection between father, mother, and child. Especially mother and child are linked by emotions; we say that their life and soul are connected. Whatever the mother wishes can manifest or be fruitful for the child. For this reason once the child has come out, the mother needs to pronounce something auspicious. Usually they say: "My dear child, you are my heart. I wish that you live a long life and see hundreds of autumns. And not only that you have a long life, but also a meaningful, joyful, and nurturing life." We consider it very important that the mother says that because, as I said, the mother's wish has a great possibility to become true for the child.

Then we need to cut the umbilical cord. Normally we measure four fingers from the baby and four from the placenta and cut in between. When we cut, it is very important not to drop the blood, so we first push the blood toward the baby, tighten the two sides and then cut in the centre. The blood in the umbilical cord is the child's blood of the soul, it has the highest power to help the immune system prevent diseases and regenerate the body system. In Tibetan medicine we have kept it since thousands of years ago. Today Western medicine also says that the placenta has this high power; so wealthy people save pieces of the umbilical cord in what they call a cord blood bank. I found it very interesting when I heard that. This shows that what the ancient healing system of the Tibetan medicine, the Himalayan knowledge, already said thousands of years ago, without any modern technology, is now being studied by millions of people who arrived at the same results. So I find it very important for the Tibetan medicine and also very interesting.

Postpartum Immediate Care

After cutting the umbilical cord the baby is separated from the placenta, so he is free. The second auspicious action is touching the outer nature, washing the baby with warm water mixed with milk and a small amount of essence of sandalwood. Sandalwood is the best medicine to prevent heat-nature diseases. It is also very good for lungs. There are two types of sandalwood: red and white. The red one is good for the blood system and the white one is good for the nervous system, even though they have the same nature.

After the washing we write the letter DHI, which is the seed syllable of Manjushri, on the tongue of the baby; we use liquid saffron as ink. Of course, we are not pulling the baby's tongue and writing on it, we just do it symbolically. Many times we have a seal with that letter, so we just touch the baby's tongue with that. In this way we are wishing that the baby has a healthy throat. Throat is the source of voice. Voice is one of the energies, which are maintaining our life. Voice is not only for singing or talking, it is also empty, and emptiness is the tool of energy. Another function of that seed syllable is for children to have success and good learning at school. Saffron is also a very powerful natural medicine for heat-nature diseases and is specially a medicine for the liver and for the whole blood system. Blood is fundamental for growing, to give energy or substances to the rest of the body. Saffron and sandalwood have a long history. When we study Tibetan herbs, each one has its own monograph, explaining why that plant has become a medicine, what is its taste, its function, its nature, which part can be used, and so on. These monographs can be quite extensive.

Also, as we said yesterday, we put on the baby a small bracelet of garlic. You know that garlic is smelly: its purpose is to protect the baby from provocations. At the same time we also put a small piece of butter with honey on the tongue of the baby. Honey and butter are both essences: one comes from plants, the other from animals' digestion; butter is also very pure because to get to that level it is digested and then divided into pure and impure. In Tibetan medicine these two substances are considered the highest nutrition we can find. Also they both have a sweet taste, so it is like introducing the first food with nonviolent nutrition essence and therefore wishing the child to live with pure essence nutrition and nonviolent food. When we present the different tastes, symbolically, sweet is positive, happy, joyful; that is why we introduce this kind of food to the child.

Then we introduce nursing, which has a few purposes. One is to nourish the baby and the other is that the sucking of the milk makes the mother's uterus shrink. Therefore nursing is very important not only for the child but also for the mother. If the uterus stays stretched for an extended period, certain air can enter, so later we have a bloating abdomen or also inflammations. So it is very important that the mother's uterus shrinks before accumulating other substances. That is why we try to nurse the baby with mother's milk as soon as possible, in order to prevent certain diseases in the mother as well. So this is about the first moments or the first days care.

Then we give the child a name. In the Tibetan tradition we get the name from two sources. One is the maternal uncle's side. In our tradition the maternal uncle is a very important person for the life of the child (I am not saying that the father's side uncle is not important, but when we give the name it is usually chosen by the maternal uncle' side). The second source of the name is the lama or the master that the family trusts or follows.

During the first three days we prefer that mother and child do not see guests and stay in a quiet place. On the third day the family and relatives perform the first ceremony to welcome the child; in the first week we have a ceremony inviting also friends, neighbors, and others.

Postpartum Nutrition

During the first six months the baby is not able to eat food. In our culture after three months we do introduce some food to him, but until the sixth month, we try to focus mainly on what the mother eats. From the sixth month on we focus more on child's food.

For the child's growth, it is very important to have food with sweet and sour tastes; dairy products are important, meat products are important too. For Tibetans it is very important to boil milk. Children especially are not allowed to drink raw milk because during childhood, as we said before, there is a lot of mucus, and milk, especially raw milk, can produce more mucus. It is not only important to boil milk, but also to put some tiny portions of honey in it, because honey has the power to absorb the mucus and keeps the lungs healthy. It also has the power to eliminate impure substances and is very good for strengthening the bones and developing the sense organs.

When we talk about meat we mean broth, soup, which is very important in the development of children. If a child does not eat meat, even though he looks healthy, very active, smart, and it seems that he is growing well, when a secondary cause happens, like a bone injury, it is harder for the bone to rebuild. The child becomes very sensitive to cold or hot, he grows very weak and, as he gets older, he has more mental problems, like anxiety, or physical problems. When the child is one year old he looks good, but in ten or twenty years what you are doing today may not prove to be the best. I am not saying that you should feed the child only meat and dairy products, balance is important.

When the child is three months old, in Tibet we do a large ritual practice to introduce him to the local guardians, sort of deities of the family. As in modern society, when a new family member is born we must go to the town hall to register him legally. We also perform a rite to the local guardians and deity protectors.

Part Two: Treatment of Diseases

We have discussed what we need to do to have a healthy child, in any case, a welcomed child. Now we talk about diseases that can manifest from the first days on. There are two conditions for a disease to manifest; one comes from the mother, the other from the child. If during the pregnancy the mother's diet and behavior were not balanced, that brings either excess, or a division, of *lung, tripa*, and *pekan.* Both conditions will affect the baby and so, since birth, the baby comes with certain diseases that in Western medicine are called genetic. So sometimes we have children with disability or some serious heart disease.

These kinds of diseases are not easy to treat and Tibetan medicine is not so good at working on this topic. Western medicine uses surgery and other techniques, with good results, and I am really grateful to see these achievements. We Tibetans put the genetic diseases under the category of the karmic diseases. So we do a lot of ritual practices or a lot of payback rites, trying to accumulate good merits.

When the illness is a condition produced by the child, three factors are involved: provocations, behavior, and diet. We will talk about provocation a little later. As far as behavior, if the person who takes care of the baby, the mother, the baby sitter, or whoever, does not pay attention and the baby falls down or something happens, it is more an injury than an illness, because at this time the baby's bones are not yet formed and are very fragile.

Regarding food, if the baby eats excessively hot or sour, or cool-nature food that is not good. Hot means spicy, but it can also refer to the nature of food. Talking about the nature of food, in the meat group for example, lamb is considered warm-heavy, chicken is cool-light, beef is neutral, pork is cool-heavy, and fish is warm-light. So, children eating too much lamb, having lamb soup every day, will accumulate warm nature in the body. If they eat too much pork, they will accumulate more heaviness. We call this a wrong diet. There is an excess or deficiency of certain substances and, as a consequence, disease will arise, so a balanced diet is important.

In the clinical practice of Tibetan medicine we have twenty-four different diseases for children: eight minor diseases, eight major diseases and eight more serious diseases. In Tibetan terms we say *trawa*, *ragpa*, and *shipa*. *Trawa* means subtle or minor; *ragpa* is more serious; and *shipa* is more specific. Today we are not going to discuss them, but we can talk about the two systems to observe a disease: the general symptoms and the specific symptoms.

The General Symptoms

The first general symptom is that the child is crying a lot. The only way for the baby to communicate is crying, because he has not developed speech yet. So, if the child is crying all the time or very strongly, that means there is something wrong. The second is if the child is trying to grab onto some parts of the body with his hands: that means he is having problems in that place. And third, if the baby becomes kind of sleepy, does not want to open his eyes, has difficulty seeing and the complexion becomes a little dull, not bright, does not play or has difficulties in breathing, the voice becomes weak, and the fingernails become longer and sharp; all this indicates that there is something wrong with him. The first series of symptoms are at the physical level, while the fact that the fingernails are sharp indicates more of a provocation disease.

Diagnosis

When we talk of diagnosis, in Tibetan medicine we have thirty-eight systems, summarized into three: observation, touching, and inquiries, or questions and answers. Concerning observation, we can look at many things, but especially we look at the tongue, the eyes and the urine. Regarding touching, we can touch various parts of the body, we check the temperature, the body's form and so forth, but mainly we take the pulse. As far as question and answer is concerned, we ask many things, but more specifically what the cause of the diseases is, where the pain is, what the symptoms are and what are the effects.

From newborn children, however, we cannot get the urine. Also we cannot check the pulse, because the rules we generally use to check the points of the pulse do not correspond in the babies as their wrists are too small for the doctor's fingers. So, until the children are eight years old, we are not able to take the pulse and what we do is read the back of the ears, where there are some very clear veins that look like the veins of a leaf. As children grow up, the ears become softer and we cannot see the veins very well, but during childhood they are very clear. The system of reading is the same, so we look at both ears and through them we read the eleven organs. Not only the eleven organs, we can also tell the strength of the baby: the physical strength, the energy strength, the life strength; there are different levels of strength we check.

Until children are three, but especially in the first year, it is difficult to collect the urine, so, instead of the baby's urine, we read the mother's milk. The explanations are the same as when we read the urine. So these are our methods for diagnosis. And then we can ask the mother what is her diet, behavior, and so on. That is how we try to identify the disease.

Most Common Diseases

One common type of childhood disease affects lungs; another affects the intestines, the digestive system. These two are the most common childhood diseases found in the clinic. There is a reason or background for why children's lungs are weak. When we talk of *lung, tripa*, and *pekan*, the three main humors, each of them has a location, a main seat. *Pekan*, or phlegm, is located in the upper part of the body, mainly in the chest. It is a combination of water and earth elements, which means it is heavy, sticky, stable, cold. Moreover, the child in the mother's womb is eating, sleeping, and especially living with the mother's womb liquid; he stays there for thirty-eight weeks eating and not moving, so he develops a lot of mucus. So once the baby comes out, he is full of heaviness. What he does then is eat and sleep; babies are basically sleeping for twenty-four hours. Why do they sleep so much? Because their nature is that of the phlegm. Then slowly they grow and sleep less and less. Once they reach old age, they are not able to sleep (many people have this problem and need sleeping pills; not sleeping is one of their many worries). Since children have a lot of mucus in the lungs, the lungs are already inflamed because they are too wet, there is too much liquid there. So, as soon as the weather changes, or in the changing seasons, like from autumn to winter, or winter to spring, children get the flu and a runny nose very easily. They cough and spit, and a lot of mucus comes out, because the *pekan* is already there. Once the weather gets damp and cold, that becomes a secondary cause to make it heavier and cooler, so the baby has more lung problems. As I said before, if you eat a small amount of honey everyday it is like a daily mucus cleaning, so the lungs are much better. That does not mean you should eat a lot of honey to clean faster. The best is to take it in the early morning, before eating, with something warm. Or at the time the baby is drinking milk you can add a little in the milk. That is about lungs. It is also good to put some white sandalwood essential oil on the chest and rub it in a little, because sandalwood has cold nature and that helps the inflammation go down.

The second common problem for children is digestion. That, too, is related to the fact that in childhood there is a predominance of *pekan*, which is cool, heavy, and sticky. Children do not yet have strong heat developed in the body. To digest food a certain heat is needed, and since in children heat is not yet developed, plus they have heavy *pekan,* that also damages the heat, it is very important that they eat warm, cooked food. And it is also important not to have too much sweet, such as cane sugar.

When we talk of sweet in Tibetan medicine, but not only in Tibetan medicine, we have three different types of sweet: honey, sugar, and molasses. Honey has a warm, light nature. Warmth has the power to melt the *pekan* and light to absorb the heaviness of things. Cane sugar is cold, heavy, so it has the power to develop more mucus and is harder to digest. Molasses is warm, heavy; it is good for the elderly because heaviness keeps the wind down. So we can simply say that honey is good for childhood, cane sugar is good for the middle age, and molasses is good for the elderly.

Children drink a lot of sweet beverages and this is not good for them when they are growing, because their digestive system is not as strong as in adults, they cannot digest everything. Since we are developed countries we have a huge selection of food and especially we have a lot of sweet things to drink and eat. Have you seen how many children are diabetic now? Diabetes is not a children's disease, it usually is a disease of old age, at least for fifty-year-old people. But today many children have diabetes and also anxiety and depression. Normally children's job is to eat and play, so ideally they should not have so much worry. Depression and anxiety are more problems of middle age people, because they work hard trying to maintain the family and have many worries. But today how many children take antidepressants? So there is something wrong. It might be that our society has undergone many changes and this is very stressful for children: maybe there are lot of things to see, to hear and that somehow affects them. It could also be the food, because food is entering our body every day. Children eat too much junk food. In Tibetan medicine, uncooked food is not nutritious: in order to get the essence of food you need to cook it. Either you cook it in a pot or in the stomach. The stomach is not designed to cook raw, heavy food. Maybe it tries to do a good job for one or two days, for one or two months but one day it gives up. As I said before, children have *pekan* nature, their digestive system is weak so it is very important to have cooked food like broth, nutritious but light to digest.

We eat, our stomach digests and then it needs a little rest. We say that normally five hours should elapse between meals: one hour for decomposing, one hour for extracting, one hour for dividing, one hour for cleaning, and one hour rest. Then it can receive the next workload. If you do not cook the food, everything needs to be done in the stomach. Then the three digestive heats [*menyam, juged, nyaged*] need to work overtime and do not have time to rest, so sometimes they delay the cleaning and gradually people become overweight because they do not digest well. They look big but in truth they are weak. Today we see this kind of problem not only in senior or middle-aged people, but in a lot of children as well.

Part Three: Provocation Diseases

The third topic is provocation diseases. Provocation is something harming, attacking. They can be visible things but normally are invisible beings. We call them *dön*. Now I will show you an image that depicts certain characters or certain symptoms from the *dön*. In general, in regard to children, we have fifteen different types of provocation diseases but twelve are more active. Five have male aspect and seven have female aspect. Provocation is translated as evil spirits. They can be evil spirits but not always; they can also be something different. As I said before, children are very easily attacked and this is for many reasons.

Provocation Symptoms

How can we find out if there is a provocation attack? Some general symptoms are if the child is crying, particularly or more often at sunset or in the late evening and yawning a lot. Children experiencing this kind of attack try to bite their lower lip; they grab at the mother and try to attract her attention. They reject the mother's nipples; become very weak and not only weak but their eyeballs are rolled up. They vomit with bubbles. When they are claiming their mother's attention and always trying to hug her, it is said that they are trying to protect themselves because they are scared of something. When they are biting their lips they are trying to show some sort of strength against that provocation. And eyeballs rolled up means they are now contaminated or strongly attacked by the provocation, so they lose consciousness. As far as crying in the late evening, at this time all human activities are slowing down and others activities are beginning, so that can also mean that other spirits are waking up now and starting to move. Also, these babies' nails are very sharp, they look like knives, when they grab somewhere you really feel it. Also, they sweat a lot. These kinds of symptoms show that a baby is having trouble with provocations.

Provocation Treatment

We have a double treatment for provocations. As we said before, when the provocations attack and the symptoms are that the children are crying and grabbing at the mother, we need to do some ritual practices to release the provocations. If there is also vomit, we need to treat the physical body. So first we need to do a ritual practice, then give some physical treatment.

Talking about ritual practices, there are two different types we can perform: peaceful and wrathful. The aim of the practice is to activate a sort of a dialogue with that spirit, trying to make it leave or become a friend. So, first we start peacefully, trying gently, kindly, asking in a gentle way to please go away, making the being understand that it is not a good idea to stay or attack this baby. That practice can be done either by a lama or I think a good practitioner can also do it.

When we talk of wrathful practice, wrathful means to threaten, like to say: "Hey, go, do not do this, this is not your territory!" so the threat is stronger. You can also understand this with logic: when you want to say something strong to someone, first you need to be a little firm, right? Otherwise, instead of you attacking the person maybe he will beat you up. In this case instead of being firm, it is better to stay quiet. So, before doing a wrathful practice you need to be a good practitioner, otherwise you make [the spirits] sort of angry without having the capacity to really overcome them. When we read or chant wrathful mantras it looks easy, but to have a real function you need a power.

As a peaceful practice, Green Tara practice is good, Vajrasattva practice is good, and any kind of a peaceful deity practice is good for protecting yourself and communicating with that being. Wrathful practices like Sinhamukha and Guru Tragphur are good; the point is that you need to be a good practitioner. Especially if you are practicing to help someone you need to be good, otherwise, instead of doing something helpful, maybe it will come back to you. Sometimes when we watch movies, we can see weak people trying to do something against the mafia but instead the mafia tortures them. So it is better not to make certain beings angry, better to stay quiet.

This is my talk for today, thank you for having listened.

If you are interested in studying Tibetan medicine, at the Shang Shung Institute of America we have ongoing courses. You can attend in person or on online. We will have a new four-year online program, starting on January 29. The four years are divided into eight semesters. Every semester you need to go where your teacher is, for a period of ten days to two weeks; the rest of the time you can follow the course online. The purpose is to make it easier for people who cannot attend the medicine program personally. Still we need to keep the essence, commitment, and quality, for this reason you need to be with the teacher for a certain time, to review things and to take the exams, so you are either promoted or not to the next year's class. You can find all information on the website of the Shang Shung Institute.

Also in September we are going to have new students of Kunye massage therapy. Kunye is not only massage, it is an external therapy of the Tibetan medicine; this course requires physical attendance with a teacher.

And then this year on May 29, we are going to have the first Tibetan medicine class in Moscow, at Kunsangar North. This project comes from the kindness of Chögyal Namkhai Norbu, to give the opportunity to people who speak Russian to study Tibetan medicine. As I said the other day, whatever we at Shang Shung Institute are doing is a project of Chögyal Namkhai Norbu and is under His leadership. So I take this opportunity to explain these things and I would also like to ask you, whatever Gar you belong to, for your support and help. Tibetan medicine is for the benefit of all sentient beings and to help sentient beings your collaboration is very important. If you need more information you can go to the Russian or American or Italian website of Shang Shung Institute, all the information is there. Thank you.

PRESENTATION

LHUSHAM GYAL
Preparation and Usage of Tibetan Herbal Medicines

January 15, afternoon

Tonight our topic is how to gather and prepare herbs. In general in Tibetan medicine, when we talk about medicines, there are three major components: animal products; herbs; and minerals. Herbs are more common. There are many Tibetan herbal books. A very famous one, called *The Necklace of Crystal*, mentions more than two thousand plants and herbs.

Part One: Gathering and Conserving Herbs

Throughout the history of Tibetan medicine and for Tibetan doctors, it has always been very important to understand and to be able to recognize all the plants and herbs. Firstly, because herbs grow everywhere, they are easy to find wherever you go. Secondly, compared to other materials herbs are very cheap. Thirdly, herbs are very easy to gather and to prepare in making up medical formulas. An understanding of the various features of herbs is thus very important for Tibetan doctors. In the *Gyüzhi* – the major Tibetan medicine textbook, translated as the *Four Tantras* – seven rules or seven principles are mentioned for herbs, and doctors need to follow these in order to be herbalists. The purpose of these seven principles is mainly to improve and maintain the quality of the medicines produced. So, the purpose of these rules is to ensure good quality herbs. We can put it like this: we strengthen the herbs so as to strengthen the formula.

What are these seven rules or seven steps of Tibetan medicine? The first is to grow the herbs in their natural habitat.

The second one is to gather them at the right time, which means that the different plants and the different parts of the medicinal plants have to be gathered in different seasons, at different times of the day, on certain special auspicious dates, and so on. All this is part of gathering at the right time.

The third step is to dry and store them well. This means, for example, that once you have gathered the herbs from the mountain, you need to know with what kind of water to rinse them, how you detoxify them, how you dry the herbs, how you store them, and so on.

The fourth principle is that once the herbs have been gathered, once you have dried and stored them, at a certain point they lose their nature, their essence, so you need to replace them. So here the texts say how long you can use the herbs, one year or two, or six months.

The fifth step is how to detoxify plants. For example, the stem of a shrub can be medicinal, but the pith, the soft part inside, may be poisonous. So we need to know how to separate this, how to divide them.

The sixth topic is to make the herbs smooth, meaning edible.

The seventh is how to formulate. So topics six and seven are not directly connected to gathering the herbs, but rather to making up medicines, the timing for the formula, how to make up a formula, how to make them edible, and how to avoid side effects.

Tonight we will be focusing more on the first five topics: where herbs grow, how to gather them, when to gather, how to dry, and how to detoxify.

The first topic is about the natural habitat of herbs. What does this mean? It means the place where certain herbs or plants need to grow.

For example, herbs with a cool nature, which treat the heat-nature ailments, need to be grown in cool climates. If they grow below 2,000 meters, for example, or in a warm-nature climate, they will not work. Some herbs need to grow at over 4,000 meters above sea level. If they grow, or we cultivate them, below 2,000 meters, then the nature of the herb, its function, will not be the same. They look as if they are the same herbs, but they work differently, because their climate was different and their cultivation was different. Similarly, if the medicine is for cool-nature ailments, made of plants like pomegranate fruit, or asafetida, for instance, if they grow in north facing or in cool climate places their function will be different. So, the pomegranate fruit grown in a south facing or a sunny warm place has a different function from when grown in a shady or cool place.

The second topic is about gathering at right time. That is based on the intended use of the herbs. You need to gather according to the part of the plant you are going to use in the medicine – the roots, or the stem, or the leaves, or the seeds. For example, roots need to be gathered in wintertime. In addition, for some medicines you have to gather in autumn and for others in summer; some in early summer and late spring. It is also very important to choose or select an auspicious date for gathering herbs. This can be chosen based on the doctor's age or by looking at certain constellation and so forth. That is in general, but sometimes there are also herbs that you can gather only on one specific day of the year. And not only on one day, but also at a specific hour. So, we do have also this kind of herb, very special herbs. Some herbs are classified according to the purpose, some herbs you have to gather in the first week of every month.

To summarize, if we use the roots, or the trunk, or the branches of a plant (in this case we are talking about certain big trees that we use in medicine), we gather them in the autumn. If it is the leaves we are going to use for the medicine, we commonly gather them in summertime. If the flowers are used in the medicine, we gather in the late summer and early autumn, in the second month of autumn at latest. It should not be too late, because otherwise the flowers disappear. Certain medicines, for example a type of rhubarb shrub, need to be gathered during wintertime. If you gather it during the other seasons, its function or power will be different.

If you are using as medicine the bark of a tree, you need to gather it in the springtime. If you gather it in the late spring, summer, or autumn, it will function differently. The time to gather the herb being used for medicine is based on its use or purpose. For example, if we are going to use the medicine as a laxative then we gather it when the energy of the plant is going down towards the roots, which means late autumn. In contrast, if we want to use it as an emetic, as the energy needs to go up to the upper gate, then we will gather it during the springtime, when the energy is surging, that is during the flowering.

In Tibetan medicine when we go to gather herbs, before we touch the plant we recite mantras such as the Medicine Buddha mantra, whose purpose is to strengthen the medicine. Another mantra we recite is the Harmonizing Mantra. Its purpose is to make everything interdependent, balanced, or harmonized; everything then becomes smooth. This means that we will not harm the land, we will do no harm to any spirits of the land and in the meantime the medicine holds its own energy. So, reciting mantras is also very important. And also prayers or saying something auspicious.

Not only this, but also we consider that the person who starts the gathering, who leads the group and first touches the herbs, needs to be a very positive person. When doctors gather herbs, first they take a shower in the morning and they wear clean clothes. But also the person who first touches herbs should have a good name, an auspicious name such as "Benefactor" (benefactor means that the medicine is going to benefit all humanity and all sentient beings). Traditionally we use children to lead this kind of thing. Children have very pure minds, and will probably not have yet performed any bad actions, thus they are very pure, and clean outside and inside.

So, as regards the second topic, gathering in time, we have discussed three aspects: how to gather herbs in general; and specifically when to gather the herbs; and the leading person.

The third topic is about proper drying after gathering. After gathering the herbs there are two very important things. The first is that you need to wash them, to rinse herbs in the same local water is very important. The second is that after you have gathered the herbs you need to soften them a little, by pounding them, or by chopping them up small. So these two are very important parts. After that, if the purpose of medicine is to treat cool-nature diseases you need to dry the herbs in the sun, in sunny sites, or outdoors on the stove, on the heat. Somehow you need to dry them by using heat. But if the purpose of the medicine is to cure heat-nature diseases, you need to dry them in a shady place or a cool, windy place. In all such cases, you need to dry them by cold nature means.

The fourth topic is about proper storage of herbs and their duration. The energy or essence of herb lasts a very short while. For example, herbs gathered in 2012 should not be used in 2013, so you need to throw them away and gather and store fresh herbs. In general it is very important to replace your herbs every year; in particular any kind of green leaf medicines and flowers *must* be replaced otherwise they will not work. The qualities of seeds, roots, and stems last a little longer.

As we said before, in Tibetan medicine formulas we not only use herbs, but also animal products and grains. Basically Tibetan medicine uses everything. Grains and animal products can be used within two or three years, because their energies last a little longer. But herbs have to be replaced each year otherwise the medicine will not work. For example, why do the herbs of some doctors function very well, while those of other doctors do not work well? Because in the first case the herbs have been replaced, in the second they may not have been changed, that is the difference. Fresh herbs, then, have more power.

The fifth topic is about detoxifying. It means that for certain rough qualities or inedible things either we cut and throw away parts or separate, or burn them; we need to do something. So, inedible substances are separated from the edible so that the edible herbs or plants can be made smoother. For example, when we talk of leaves as medicine, if there are things like thorns or hairs on the leaves, those are the poisonous things that we need to take out. If the medicinal plant itself is a poisonous plant, we need to detoxify it either with a system of burning, or cooking or by mixing it with other medicines in order to detoxify it. There are many ways, but the important thing is that they are detoxified. We focus on the detoxifying stage mainly during the preparation stage. Most information is included when we prepare the medicine, during the formula stage. Later I will explain this topic in more depth.

The sixth topic is about processing the herbs, what in Tibetan we refer to as making them "smooth." Whatever needs to be detoxified we detoxify and then the herb is made smooth or edible. And not only this. It also includes the concept of the formula and how to prepare the medicine.

The seventh topic is based around the illness to be treated: which kind of tastes we need to mix together, the nature of the medicine we need to mix together, and which kind of post-digestion medicine we need to put in the mixture. So the seventh topic basically concerns how to make medicine or formulations according to the particular ailment to be treated. The last two topics, then, are not directly connected to the gathering, but more to making formulas.

Part Two: How to Make Formulas

When we talk about how to formulate, we also talk about how to detoxify or how to prepare medicines. The preparation of medicines is a very important part of how to use herbs. Indeed, some herbs, with a certain formula, a certain detoxifying process, a certain kind of preparation, are used for stomach diseases but if we change the detoxifying system, the same herbs then become good for the small intestine; and if we add something or we take away something then they become good for gynecological problems. Even if it is the same main ingredient, the detoxifying method, or the way the formula is prepared changes the function of the medicine. For this reason it is very important to understand the system and how to formulate.

The second purpose of *duljon* – which means to make a formula or to make smooth – is that the medicine should be easy to digest. Easy to digest means that it can get more quickly to the problem and also produce more benefit, a full benefit. This is the second purpose of carrying out detoxification or to make and prepare formulas.

Now we will go more specifically into how we carry out the detoxification and how we make herbs smoother. When we use roots for a medicine, the outer bark of the root is poisonous, so we need to remove it.

If the stem is to be used for the medicine, inside the stem there is something white, soft, it looks like foam: that, too, is poisonous and needs to be taken out, to be cleaned.

If the medicine involves using a branch, between branches there are joints: the joint is poisonous, so we need to take it out or to clean it.

If a leaf is to be used for the medicine, the stems of the leaves are poisonous. They must be taken off or cleaned.

If the flower of a plant is to be the medicine, the sepals are poisonous, so we need to take them out or clean them.

If the fruit is to be the medicine, inside the fruit there is a hard bit that we call bone: that is poisonous and we need to take it out.

These are the general rules when using herbs. Then, specifically, there are also herbs that need to be cooked in water, or to be roasted or fried on the stove.

A general, but very important rule for detoxifying with water, as I said before, is that you need to rinse or wash the herbs with water from the same valley, region, or village where you gathered them. Certain herbs need to be left in water for a minimum of twenty minutes to a maximum of six or seven hours. Some herbs not only need to be soaked in water, but also to be cooked in water like asparagus, for example. Some herbs, like seeds, need to be left soaking in milk if used for certain purposes, or sometimes in blood. These are the medicinal ingredients that need detoxifying in water, but there are also herbs that need to be detoxified by fire.

Detoxifying in fire does not mean to put the herbs directly on the fire, but rather in a ceramic container that we seal well and then put on the fire in the charcoal. It is a sort of long-term slow cooking like when making ash. For example, in the case of rhododendron, which is either used for the stomach or for the joints, we need to detoxify it with fire: not in direct contact with fire, but rather sealed in a container. Certain medicines also need to be fried in a pot. Some plants we just cook, some need to be cooked with sand or other substances: we heat up the sand and put the medicine into the sand so they are kind of roasted.

For example, how do we detoxify rhubarb? We first soak it in wine to make it a little fresh or wet; then we cook it in a dry frying pan.

Thorns and this kind of thing we roast in sand. This way they do not enter into contact with the dry pot, but are roasted and detoxified in the sand.

How do we detoxify castor seeds? The castor seed is a poisonous plant; we detoxify it by roasting the seeds in barley flour. First we heat the barley flour, then we put in the seeds and roast them together. In this way the medicine has more power to function as a laxative.

Certain medicines need not only to be cooked in water, but also to be steamed in order to be detoxified. An example is the leaves or stems of the rhubarb.

The last topic I would like to present is how to make a paste. Pastes in Tibetan medicine are very important. Their purpose is to strengthen the nature or the quality of the medicine. The medicine itself thus becomes very soft and more edible, with no poison.

In general, we can make a tincture or paste (paste means that the nature is concentrated) with any kind of herb or plant. In ancient times we used to use deer musk for certain medicines, to cure infections or inflammation, but today the use of animal products is less common, we do not often use animal products now. For this reason, when we need a medicine for infections or inflammation, we use a plant that is very effective for infections (sorry, I do not remember the English name; in Tibetan we call it *chabuba*) and make a tincture or paste. It is more or less equivalent to deer musk.

Juniper is high on the list of plants used for medicines in Tibetan formula. We use juniper berries, juniper roots, juniper leaves, and so forth. But we can also make juniper paste. In this case its function or power increases, it doubles, or triples. That helps to strengthen the life, strengthen the sense organs, and extend life. And this paste is also very good to strengthen the soul. So, when these herbs are made into paste, that helps to strengthen the nature of the plant and the plant or herb become doubly, triply powerful.

Medicine, which has been detoxified, is made more edible and smooth – smooth means with fewer side effects. Herbs should first of all have strong power and function, and secondly they should not have strong side effects. For example, in general, laxatives are good for certain illnesses, but they can also be quite harmful for the body. So when we make medicine with ingredients for a laxative, as we have discussed before, using castor seeds, we then detoxify and make it into a paste, so then they work better than the raw plant, but without harming the body.

What I have explained now is how using raw herbs in medicine is different from making a sort of paste: the function is different and the side effects are different. This is not something I am just saying or my opinion, it has been clinically proved. When we use a laxative, if the herbs or ingredients are not detoxified, or not made into a paste, they do have the laxative function, causing diarrhea, but at the same time the person will also have vomiting, or pain and afterwards will lose appetite, weight, and so on. So, there are other problems, other side effects. But if we use the medicines in paste form, and use this as a laxative, they work better, and so then you can use very small dose:

the function is the same, but they do not have side effects like vomiting or pain, or loss of appetite.

If you take a non-detoxified medicine, its nature is a little rough, which means that it is both difficult to digest, and also it does not have the function it is supposed to have. That is why we say it is poisonous, but this does not mean that if you eat it today you will die tomorrow, we are not talking about poison like a chemical poison.

That is my presentation for today. Thank you for your listening and participation. I would like to leave a few minutes for questions. Thank you.

Q: What do you mix the herbs with to make paste?

A: We just mix the herbs with water and then boil, make kind of decoction and then make the paste. But we need to regulate the heat according to the plant or herbs. They do not all need the same level of heat.

Q: How is Chinese medicine different from Tibetan medicine?

A: We often get this kind of question. My humble answer is, first, I did not study traditional Chinese medicine, so for me to say it is this or that is a little hard. But based on the results of my research, it seems certain things are different.

One example is that of the use of the licorice herb. In Tibetan medicine we use licorice for illnesses of the *lung*, or special excess heat in the lungs, or a lung infection. It seems that traditional Chinese medicine more commonly uses licorice for stomach and other diseases. That is a little different.

To give you another example, in Tibetan medicine, as I said before, we have many ways to make up formulas. Firstly, we make a formula based on taste. Secondly, a formula is based on the function of the medicine. Thirdly, formula is based on the post-digestion taste. So, our formulas have many levels, a rough level and a more final or subtle level. It seems that you will not find this in traditional Chinese medicine. But as I said before I did not study Chinese medicine, and for me it is hard for me to say yes or no.

Q: In Tibet do people actually know the benefits of plants, are they able to cure themselves by using them, or do they need to go visit a doctor and ask for advice?

A: It is not very common for people to know how to gather herbs by themselves and how to make medicines by themselves. Mostly yes, when they are sick they need to see a doctor. But some village people help doctors every year, go with a doctor to gather herbs. This kind of person will know about herbs, after they have followed the doctor gathering herbs for many years. So, when they are sick they may know how to gather something and how to make a decoction and drink or eat the medicine, that kind of thing.

PRESENTATION

KUNCHOK GYALTSEN
Geriatrics in Tibetan Medicine

January 16, morning

Today the subject is the care of elders. When we speak of older people it is awkward, because everybody wants to be young. In Tibet if we say "You look older" people would be happy. I do not know if this is true in Europe, but in America if you say, "You look older" that is considered unfortunate.

In Tibetan medicine the way the care of older people is presented in textbooks is mainly rejuvenation of the physical body through spiritual practice. Even though we use rejuvenation pills, employing medicinal herbs to make what we call *chüdlen,* the spiritual practice is more important. Since we are talking about the care of the elder in the West, I will try to compare your cultural situation in terms of the division of children, younger adults, and older people in Tibetan medicine. About the elderly, the *Mennag Gyüd,* which is the third part of the *Gyüzhi,* says that before sixteen years of age people are regarded as children; after sixteen until seventy we consider them *tarma* or adults, which signifies having a stronger body. After seventy people are *genba* which means older.

I think the consideration of old age is similar in today's modern society because you retire at sixty-five. Society also knows you have become older and therefore less capable physically, so you are asked to stop work.

Today I do not want to share the many techniques of how to take care of the elderly, but wish to explain how we view age, as that could be helpful for you. Before you can take care of yourself, a right attitude toward aging needs to be determined. When I was in the United States of America, I felt strongly that many people want to be younger and that the society itself tends to favor young people. People wear colorful clothes, for example, try to look young, and apply a lot of makeup. Wealthy people even have operations, cosmetic surgery, and do a large amount of exercise in an effort to be young. That is actually a little sad because once we reach a certain age, it is very hard to act like the young because our physical body is on the way to exhaustion after many years of life.

In Tibetan society it is a compliment when we say someone is older because that statement has many aspects. One thing it indicates is that you are wiser; that you have more knowledge, and that you are in charge of many things. A lot of young people respect the old. Respect does not mean flattery, like saying, "Oh, you look so young" or "You are so active," but in their heart they always think, "Oh, he is older, so I must take care of him or her."

People who are getting older accept in their hearts the changes in their physical body. I want to emphasize that a little bit more. In Tibet people believe this particularly because of the Buddha's teaching: every human being and every sentient being has *chi ga na kye*, birth, aging, sickness, and death. Buddha said those are the Four Sufferings. It is the nature of human beings to have the Four Sufferings. First of all we must understand human nature in depth. Firstly, all objects on this earth are temporary; this is also translated as impermanent, which means always changing. There is nothing except the blue sky that is not changing; that is what impermanence means. That is why in the

Buddha's teaching there is the middle path called *uma*, and much is said about *tongpanyi* and *mitagpa*, which signify emptiness and imperma-nence. This concept helps us to understand the nature of our physical body. For example, from the moment our mother gives birth to us, we experience change: each minute, each hour, each day. Then we grow up into teenagers, adults, and then elders. Our hair became gray and falls out, we become wrinkled, lose teeth, our eyesight becomes bad: all this is a natural development or change.

In Buddhist teaching emptiness does not mean empty in the nor-mal sense; the meaning has to do with the truth that not one time or one place can be found that is not always changing. Because there is always change and difference, any phenomenon can be regarded as empty. Those concepts are important because Buddhist monks and nuns usually practice *dagme*, selflessness, as in trying to find what in your body is actually you: are you always present or are you always changing, where is this "you"? You have to realize that, and it is a very important practice. When you understand that, you understand the nature of all existence and then it does not matter that things change or that you get older.

Getting older, we all face the suffering of fear. For example, when you look in the mirror and see that ten years ago you were younger and now you are older, sometimes you feel unhappy, seeing more wrinkles, gray hair, and so forth. Then you look at your grandchildren and at the young people in the street, and you feel upset. Do not think in that way. Look at those children or younger people with the concept of emptiness in mind: after ten years they will no longer be the same, because they also will be changed. We are not able to see that at every moment there is change, but only notice at certain times, because our wisdom or our eyes are limited in understanding. If we understand *dagme* well and you have realized it, then you can grasp that every moment changes.

That we have birth and afterward we have death means that some-thing that has a beginning has an end. Like this conference, this cultural event, for example: on the 11th we came, everybody fresh and joyful, and today we are leaving. We had a wonderful time on this island of Tenerife and now we must leave, although this leaving is actually the beginning of another chapter and new exciting experiences. That is the nature of human beings. What we call existence is always changing. That is why every moment is the end but also the beginning: we start with birth, then become older, and finally aged. Looking around us on the street or on the beach, we see so many young people full of energy. They cannot know what an old person feels, what it is like not being able to walk or having a head full of grey hair, because they have not yet had those experiences.

We are lucky to have such experiences first. It is like you are in line in a cafeteria: everybody is hungry, but you are in front, and get to the food before the others, and eat first. All those people are waiting, but you are the lucky one who is at the head of the line. With this attitude we will never feel sad to get older. Not only people getting older, but also the whole society, as well as younger people, needs to understand this. If we do not understand the nature of our condition, we cannot have a healthy society. We always talk about equality: actually having this point of view also has to do with equalization. With this understanding everyone has his or her own position and does not compete for the same spot. Then our society will be more harmonious and mutual respect for one another will arise.

All of you are interested in health. Regarding health many things can be actively done to change yourself, but in many other regards we are passive. The passive aspects also need to be changed. Once you change the passive situation, for example, those many matters in which society still needs to hold a correct view, then we can have a good environment for the aged. Otherwise if everyone wants to act like a young person, then what role can older people have? They will not have space to live out their lives, that is the problem. Many things maybe neither you nor I can change individually, but all together we can make changes. After you have understood how things should be, you should encourage those situations in your community. I think the traditional Hispanic society has this concept, but modernization forces us into a different mode, which often is not really suitable and does not fit our situation. We must understand this very carefully and then we can deal better with the situation.

Aging is a terrible thing for everybody but death is even more terrible. If you cannot deal with your aging, with getting old, how can you deal with your death? Doctor Phuntsog will hold a seminar explaining hospice care, the situation and concept of death, after death, and all related matters, so perhaps you should attend it to learn more about how those concepts are viewed in Tibetan medicine and Buddhist philosophy. Many people think that we finish at death and there is nothing more. This is very sad. Until we die we want to be tremendously active, we want to be young, and so forth. That is actually very narrow-minded, since much more than that is going on and happening.

As I said, when there is a beginning there is an end, and when there is an end there is a beginning. Our life is not one life, but many lives. That we can understand logically, since how can things be logical only at a certain time and then logic disappears entirely? That does not make sense. When we have birth, then there is death, and if there is death, then there is birth. Therefore the concept of reincarnation makes sense. Inside China many people do not believe in reincarnation and make jokes about Tibetans. Sometimes Tibetans work slower than Chinese in the cities, so that the Chinese say, "Oh you are Tibetans, you work slowly: that is okay for you because you have another life, but we do not!" It is like *mañana* here in Spain. Relatively, this tells us that Tibetan people have more understanding about what is going to happen in the future. If in your early life you do not do well, you try to do so in later life. If in your later life you cannot do better, you aim to do so in your next life. Thus you have a long-term goal and a short-term goal and can appreciate each moment of your life.

As our body changes we must think of the positive outcome associated with that change. For example, if our physical body changes, our mind is changing too. Young people make immature decisions, but as you get older, you develop strong opinions and greater wisdom and can make decisions wisely. When you have this attitude everything becomes easier. Taking *chüdlen*, using medicinal herbs, improving your diet, and behaving in an appropriate way: all these changes will be useful and helpful. Otherwise we can be disappointed, because if our understanding does not have this foundation, nothing, including the *chüdlen*, will work.

I think this kind of concept is not in conflict with other religious concepts. You need to work hard to wisely integrate this concept so that it makes sense to yourself. For example, many people do not want to grow old, and many people do not want to die. Not only today, but also many years ago people were like that. Almost two thousand years ago the king of a very powerful kingdom in China, Qin Shi Huang, did not want to die; he had conquered all of China and wanted to be its king forever. He sent envoys to the East to find longevity pills, but did not succeed in reaching his goal, and after three generations his kingdom was defeated. During the time of his kingdom he was the most powerful ruler. If you go to China, you will understand. He built a wall that crossed the whole country called The Great Wall.

If even that sort of person could not deal with aging and death, how can people like us change anything? That is why first of all you must find the right attitude toward aging. In reality we actually act in a variety of appropriate ways regarding the outdated. For example, we change numerous things: we change our clothes after a few days, and we buy new clothes over the years, because when clothes are older, we get rid of them. We buy a car, drive it for several years, and then buy another one. We change many things, but we never think about changing our physical body. We need to work on this point: the principle is the same, so we must accept it.

As I said, our body eventually exhausts itself. Many concepts exist about this, so it is difficult to explain everything here, but there are many reasons that determine the length of our lives. For example, my lifespan may be sixty years, or eighty, or one hundred. That depends on how much *le* – *le* means karma – I created, how much fortune I created. The same is true for everybody. That is why in Tibetan we call it *tsei tse*. *Tsei* means life, *tse* means limit. Everyone has that kind of lifespan. It is the same with a light bulb: when technicians design it, they establish how many hours it will last. After a certain time the bulb goes out permanently. It must end because that was its life span. The same is true for our bodies.

Earlier I said that after the age of seventy years we consider a person old, but it is not that we suddenly become old. That actually starts at birth, since we are changing every moment, little by little. That is why it depends how "old" is defined. In Tibetan medicine actually the mind and the body go in opposite directions. When you are younger, the mind is immature and then develops more and more. The physical body is stronger when you are younger, and then becomes weaker and weaker. There are many symptoms of this. In Tibetan medicine we say that *lung, tripa,* and *pekan* change the physical body, and when the *lung, tripa,* and *pekan* are exhausted, the shape of the body changes and the force or energy of the body weakens.

Also the five senses get weaker. For example, eyesight becomes poor; taste is not so acute; and tactile perception, in Tibetan *regja,* is also less sensitive. The sense of smell lessens and that of hearing diminishes. As you know, *lung, tripa,* and *pekan* have five aspects; the other day we described them. *Tripa dang giu* makes the skin thinner. Becoming more fragile, the skin becomes less colorful and less attractive and also more wrinkles appear on the face. Other examples are that the flesh will be flabby and the thinking slower. Those are the typical signs, universal symptoms that everyone develops.

When anyone gets older and still looks like a child, it is very dangerous, very bad. You should think that the signs of aging look great. If there were one hundred people above the age of seventy and we were talking about senior concerns, eating together, or whatever, and then suddenly one person became very young, like a seven-year-old boy or girl, everybody would be frightened; he or she would be like ET, a strange person.

Once we have understood what an elderly human being is, we can live longer, and although our life span is fixed, we can develop good fortune and create positive karma to make our life last longer. We do a Buddhist practice like Dzogchen so that we can understand the nature of the universe and then practice how to manage our ignorance, anger, and attachment and how to become more compassionate: all this will cause you to have a longer life. Anyone who is a very healthy person and has a very strong mind can make good choices of food, for example, and can practice many things to better life and make it last longer.

In Tibetan medicine older people have more *lung* disorder since their nature is *lung*. Thus it is necessary to think about the food you eat in taking care of *lung* disorders. Through practice and food you can take good care of your stomach: that is the foundation. When your stomach and digestion are good, oily food, a little rich and sweet, are usually positive for older people. For example butter, particularly a little aged butter – fresh butter is best for *tripa* – is good for the old. There is a sweet called *buram* [molasses] in Tibetan that is also very good. White onion is good and milk, particularly warm milk, is good. Probably the *tsampa* eaten on this island is also good.

Our president of Arura, Dr. Otsang Tsokchen, did some research on old people in Tibet. Two years ago a woman passed away who was 118 years old. She did not remember how many generations there had been in her family. She was slight and in very good health. Doctors had been visiting her every two years over a long period of time. Her diet was *tsampa*, Tibetan butter tea, and some *buram*. She often repeated that she liked those foods very much. Maybe she had the right attitude in her life. At that high altitude very simple food, and particularly those foods, are good for *lung*, so she remained in good health. She was actually from Lhokha, which is south of Lhasa. Among meats, lamb is good, although I do not know if you eat lamb here. Also beef and chicken are good for *lung*. In Tibet people make soup with bones; bones are excellent for the *lung* disorder, and thus good for aging people.

Many old people have trouble in sleeping. To sleep well during the night, you need to eat a little heavy or oily food for dinner, which will permit successful rest. In the West you drink milk and eat yogurt probably in the morning. Try to eat yogurt and drink milk in the evening before you go to sleep: one hour before bedtime, drink one glass of warm milk – usually cow's milk is good. Also you should sometimes eat yogurt, preferably a natural full fat yogurt, and then you will sleep well.

In terms of behavior, there is not much new to share with you. Actually, care of the old in public health advice also gives the same counsels. For example older people need company when they go somewhere. They need to be careful and should not go out during the night in the dark. Also sharp objects should not be left around the house. I think that you already know about this kind of advice, so it is not necessary to say much to you in this regard.

Sleep is very important: try to sleep seven to eight hours per night, although that is difficult for many people. What you can do is to take a nap during the day, particularly in springtime. In spring the body is weak. In Tibet, for example, also animals are weak in that season. We need a lot of rejuvenation then; we need to energize people and also animals. Thus in spring take more naps than in other seasons. Preparing a room for sleep is also very important: darken it a little. The walls should not be of a light color, but instead a maroon or blue color or another dark hue. Your bed should not be next to the window, but in shadow. You need to be warm; if you are warm and comfortable, you will sleep better.

If you are heavier – heavy means you have more *pekan* – you can do some exercise, but not so much. Old people should do only a little exercise. You do need to take naps, but before you take a nap do not exercise. For example, have a meal. There is very good soup in the West, like French onion soup. That kind is excellent. Eat that sort of food, some chicken, boiled or roasted, and then take a nap. Exercise after napping because after exercise you cannot sleep.

Then you need to bathe or take showers. At least once a week it is very important to clean your hair and nails and wash at minimum your feet and hands. Some old people when they get older do not wear much make-up and are very clean. That is a positive attitude. There are many elderly people whose faces are very pleasant. Other frustrated or angry elders think wrinkles are bad and put on heavy make-up. They talk in a frustrated way. They are ugly to look at. I think you should be in the first category.

As regarding medicine, use *chüdlen* medicine to energize. I do not have much information here to share with you. The composition of *chüdlen* is complex. It is a little difficult for me to explain because it requires a lot of background and preparation, and is a technical matter. In the future if you are interested, make your requests to Doctor Phuntsog Wangmo of the Shang Shung Institute Medical School. In the future maybe we can create a serious seminar, workshops, and talks in order to present more of *chüdlen* practice.

There are two kinds of *chüdlen*. One is *chüdlen*, the other is called *rotsa*. Actually they are similar and have a similar concept, but *chüdlen* is used more to rejuvenate the physical body. If you think, "I want to be the most beautiful person, the most handsome person, so I take *chüdlen*," that is a wrong motivation. Why did Tibetan masters create so many kinds of *chüdlen*? Because they wanted to extend their lives and do positive practice, like Buddhist methods to develop more com-passion: that is why the physical body needs to be stronger, the number one motivation. The second reason is that we are so busy and preparing food takes much time. Every day we prepare meals three times, we buy food, prepare it, eat, and go to the bathroom: all those things eat up our time. So the lamas created the *chüdlen* pills.

There are many kinds of *chüdlen*. When you practice *chüdlen* you do not need to eat: you can then practice twenty-four hours a day and use your time perfectly. Of course during the day everybody works, but during the night there is sleep yoga. Those techniques are used to make our lives more meaningful and effective. Many materials are used in *chüdlen*, for example stones in *do* mineral *chüdlen*. *Metog chüdlen* is a flower *chüdlen*; and then there is medicinal *chüdlen*, and another called *lung chüdlen*. So those are different *chüdlen* methods.

About one hundred years ago in Amdo a lama called Geshe Gangwa practiced *do chüdlen* and for twelve years he stayed in the mountains and never saw people. When I was young I followed my teacher to the mountains where he was in retreat and I accompanied him. Geshe Gangwa lived there for twelve years not eating any normal food, only doing *do chüdlen*. One of my teacher practiced *metog chüdlen*, *chüdlen* with nonpoisonous flowers. He picked the flowers, dried them, made pills, and then used them. At the beginning he took several pills a day, then reduced the number, diminishing little by little, until at the end he took maybe one pill a day, and he did meditation, all those things. For some kinds of *chudlens* more practice is needed, others lay people can practice. In the future we would like those teachings to be given seriously, so maybe you can request them and we can organize.

With your mind you can meditate, do prayers, and mantras. For example, before you take a nap, sit quietly and rest, reciting mantras; then nap, so you are calm and relaxed. After a good rest you will be in a very good mood. When you receive young people or anyone else, you will share friendly talk, you will smile, and people will like you and find you wonderful.

Because our time is limited, this is all for today. I wish you all the best and that you will be looking well and feeling healthy!

CONCLUDING REMARKS

NAMKHAI NORBU

January 16, morning

Good morning everybody. We are very happy to have successfully concluded this Tibetan event, specifically the one about Tibetan medicine. It has been really special because we had very important guests this year. The collaboration between the Shang Shung Institute and the Arura in Qinghai Province will continue, which means we will continue to develop for the future.

I would like to particularly thank our guests. I would also like to thank the people who organized, worked, and collaborated on this event. Finally I would like to thank the local people for their participation, this is something very important.

Phuntsog Wangmo
Good morning. It is a very happy moment. Under Chögyal Namkhai Norbu and his wife Rosa Tolli Namkhai leadership we have very successfully finished this event, which officially should have ended tomorrow. This is due to my mistake: I thought the event started on the 10th and finished on the 16th, so I gave this information to the doctors and they booked their air tickets with these dates. When I found out that it

was not so, it was too late to change their tickets. That is why the doctors need to leave today in the afternoon. Please, forgive me for my fault.

Anyway, everything went very well. I just want to thank everybody, especially the translators and all the Community supporters, the Gakyil of Barcelona and the Gakyil of Tenerife. Also I would like to thank the Shang Shung team and of course the technicians who made it possible for people to participate all over the world.

Now, on behalf of the doctors, who brought some gifts from Tibet for people here, I am going to distribute them. First to the team of translators because we need their good voice to translate in the future.

This I would like to present to the Barcelona Gakyil: thank you for your help, we need your continued support.

And this to the Tenerife Gakyil. I know that organizing this kind of event is not so easy, it is very hard work, but you have done it for the third time very successfully, so we would like you to continue.

And this I would like to present to the event team with many thanks for all your hard work.

Thanks to everybody.

Conference at ULL Pyramid Conference Hall

PROF. CHÖGYAL NAMKHAI NORBU
Death According to Tibetan Medicine

January 17, evening

Professor Alfonso M. García Hernández, PhD, Head of the Department of Nursing, University of La Laguna and President of SEIT – Sociedad Española e Internacional de Tanatologia (Spanish and International Society of Thanatology):

Good evening. Thank you for your presence. I am going to be brief. We are glad to have here once again Chögyal Namkhai Norbu, a meditation master who has visited us on various occasions in the past. We thank him for his visit this time in the name of the institution that is hosting us. In particular, I thank him as a member of the Religious Studies Group of the University of the Canary Islands. I also thank my friend Professor Francisco de Velasco, through whose auspices the pleasure of this meeting was made possible.

The Master, a professor, researcher, and much more, will speak today on the very interesting topic of death, focusing on this topic according to Tibetan medicine. It is a special subject for me as it has been one of my main focuses in recent years. The important topics about life, I would say, are mainly three: daily life, love, and death. Therefore I invite you all to participate and listen attentively and to meditate on the understanding of death according to the Tibetan approach. Thank you very much. Now I pass the word to Chögyal Namkhai Norbu.

Chögyal Namkhai Norbu:

Good evening everybody. I am sorry I am not fluent in the Spanish language, but I will try to explain and do my best in English which is, in any case, much more understandable than if I were to speak in Tibetan. These past days, the Third Tibetan Cultural Event has been taking place here, with particular concentration on Tibetan medicine and with the kind participation of important Tibetan doctors from China, Qinghai Province.

Our subject today is *The Tibetan Book of the Dead*, and that knowledge is related to Tibetan medicine. Discussing the topic of death is complex because we can neither judge nor think logically about it. When someone is dying we do not know what is happening. In a matter where logic is applicable, we can study, we can learn, and we can distinguish between what is true and what is not true based on direct or indirect logic. The subject of death, on the other hand, is very much related also to the spiritual path. We consider that through a spiritual path one develops clarity. When we ask what happens when someone dies, we need this kind of clarity to understand. Therefore, besides its link to medicine, this knowledge is connected to the spiritual path.

You know already that *The Tibetan Book of the Dead* has become extremely famous in the Western world. Originally this teaching was taught by Guru Padmasambhava, a master who in the eighth century arrived in Tibet from India. It is connected both with medicine and the spiritual path. This series of teaching in general is called Shitro in Tibetan. *Shi* means peaceful, *tro* means wrathful. What do wrathful and peaceful mean here? They are connected with the condition of the individual. For example, our nature has a calm state, but it also has the aspect of movement: the wrathful aspect manifests as movement, whereas when there is no movement we are in a calm state. This is our condition.

How can we understand this? It is not necessary that we believe a book or someone's explanation: we can observe ourselves. For example, when you think, "I have a mind," you know what mind is: mind is thinking and judging. You may ask yourself what the mind is like. When thoughts arise if you try to discover where they are and how they look, you will find that as you observe a thought, the thought disappears and you cannot find anything: this is emptiness or the calm state. Why is it we cannot find the thought? Because we have entered our real condition, which is emptiness. This does not mean that you always remain in emptiness, because immediately another thought arises. You then have the thought, "I am searching, but I cannot find where the thought is or what it is." That is another thought. Observe that thought as well: you still cannot find anything and you are again in a state of emptiness. This is our condition: the alternation of emptiness and movement. On the spiritual path to know what our real condition is, we use this method that is named after its peaceful and wrathful aspects. In a teaching, first we need to discover. After discovering, we need to possess that knowledge concretely, not only for dying but also for living.

We have three moments in our life: birth, life, and death. This is everybody's condition. We do not observe or think much about these matters. For example at a birth we are so happy, "Oh, our child is born!" But when there is birth, together with it death also appears. Although it may not occur immediately, one day somehow it will manifest because we are living in time and time is passing, time is impermanent. Even if we say that someone has a long life, maybe one hundred years, thinking that one hundred years is very long, we need to remember how centuries and centuries have passed in our history. This is the real condition. For that reason it is important for everybody to know about how our death should and must be. We are always concerned about life and what we do in it, but most people do not think that death also exists and some feel afraid, saying, "I cannot think of death otherwise I become paranoid and upset." It is not sufficient that we try not to feel badly: the time of death is coming and one day it will manifest. There is no reason to feel afraid, but we must understand how it is. This concerns not only death, but everything in our life.

Many people in their lifetime are constantly worried, thinking, "This is good, this is bad," always concentrating on good and bad. Of course in our life good and bad always exist, and it is important that we know that and live accepting that is just how it is; there is no reason for us to feel afraid. We live in time and there exists good but also bad: they always alternate. Not only the positive exists, nor only the negative. If we know this and accept it, we do not load ourselves with tensions; when problems manifest, we do our best. We must not concentrate only on our numerous problems and unfortunate circumstances, because in our existence it is also important that we relax and enjoy life.

Many people say they cannot relax since they do not know how. Why do we not succeed in relaxing? Because we give everything too much importance. We think this is important, that is important. But in a real sense nothing is important, everything is relative. For example, someone says, "Oh, today I have an important meeting and I absolutely must be there at ten o'clock." This person charges himself up and in order to get there by ten o'clock drives too fast on the road and has an accident. He can also die. Even if he does not die, he is taken to the hospital. If it is true that the meeting is so important and he must be there, why does he go to the hospital now, instead of to the meeting? A concretely important matter, you see, does not really exist. Everything is relative, but by giving a matter too much importance, we charge ourselves and develop tensions. In our lifetime it is important to relax, knowing that everything is relative. Of course, when we know that something important needs to be done we do our best, but in a relaxed way and then life goes better.

If we know that one day death will come and have that fact a little present, we can prepare ourselves. Preparation is related to knowledge and understanding. For example, this famous book *The Tibetan Book of the Dead* gives us information, allowing us to understand how death manifests. We must understand about this during our lifetime; it is insufficient that only when we are dying someone passes on this advice to us. For example, in our lifetime we have day and night. In the nighttime we fall asleep. When we fall asleep we have dreams, sometimes good, sometimes bad, until we awaken. They are connected with our mind. After death our physical body is taken to the cemetery, but our mind does not finish there. It is similar when we fall asleep: when we sleep our body lies comfortably on the bed, but then the mind wakes up and we have dreams. In dreams the function of mind is not connected with our sense organs. In the daytime, for example, to see something we open our eyes; for hearing we need to use our ears, and so forth; we are totally dependent on our sense organs. If no organs of senses existed, we would have no possibility to see or hear. This is the capacity of our physical level.

In dreaming we do not use our sense organs. In the dream state, the function of our mind is called the mental body. Here, body does not mean the physical level but refers to a dimension, the dimension of the mind, because all the senses are functioning. The function of senses combined with the mind is called the mental body. It is the same thing not only when we are sleeping but also when we are dying. In *The Tibetan Book of the Dead,* the *Bardo Thodrol* is widely explained. *Bardo* means intermediate state. In the same way, when we are falling asleep until we wake up, that state is also a kind of small *bardo*. If in our lifetime we have an understanding of our sleeping state, of dreaming, and so forth, we can also understand the after-death state. For this reason, we divide meditation practices into practices of the day and practices of the night. Practice of the night does not mean that we do not sleep and chant mantras or do visualization. What it does mean is that we do something to become aware of dreams. Becoming aware of dreams we can understand what our situation is, the dimension of the dream. If we have that awareness, we become familiar with how it will be when we die, because sleeping and dying are similar. For example, when we fall asleep, our senses of seeing and hearing gradually stop functioning; we call that "falling asleep." Falling asleep is just an example to make it easier to understand the state of death.

We divide the state of death in different *bardos* and thus can understand each of them. This explanation and knowledge is called *The Tibetan Book of the Dead*. The Western world had heard of *The Egyptian Book of the Dead*, and for that reason when *The Tibetan Book of the Dead* appeared many scholars discovered similarities and became interested. The Tibetan culture and knowledge includes not only this book on the subject of death, but also many different series of teachings called the *Shitro*. *The Tibetan Book of the Dead*, which is diffused in the Western world, is a teaching of Guru Padmasambhava. He had hidden this teaching for the future. It was discovered in 1365 by the *tertön* Karma Lingpa, who became famous as a result. *Tertön* means someone who discovers a hidden teaching. Later, in Sikkim, a Tibetan scholar called Kazi Dawa Samdup who knew English quite well was the first to translate Guru Padmasambhava's book. It was later edited by Professor W.Y Evans-Wentz, well-known in England, and published in 1927 by the Oxford University Press. Since that time this book has became celebrated. Through study and research, we have found that this translation is not one hundred percent accurate, but that is not a problem. What is important is that it was the first edition of that work introduced in the Western world and it became very famous.

This book explains the various *bardos* that correspond to all conditions. *Bardo* does not mean only a state after death: it means intermediate state. Also in this moment we are in the *bardo*. Our present dimension is called in Tibetan the Kyeshi Bardo. *Kye* means birth, *shi* means death. From birth until death we grow, we learn, we study, and so forth; all of life takes place during the state of this Kyeshi Bardo. If you are interested to know how the after-death state is and what happens in that situation, it is important to learn and become familiar with all the *bardos* while we are in this present one.

Maybe many of you have already read *The Tibetan Book of the Dead*, which says that after death we can have many different kinds of visions, wrathful, peaceful, and so forth. Not only books, but many videos and films about the *bardo* have been produced that illustrate various wrathful and peaceful manifestations. Some people have asked me, "In the East, the many peaceful and wrathful deities and manifestations are precisely related to their cultures. As Westerners, we do not have an Eastern culture and so how can we have these visions?" You should know that these visions are not culture-related. Being from the East, for example a Tibetan, a Chinese, or an Indian, and having that culture does not imply that when the person dies he or she will experience these visions that are related strictly to individual potentiality. In this lifetime if you have received the transmission of this teaching and learned about it, then you have the possibility of experiencing these manifestations. If you have never received this teaching, its transmission, or knowledge of it during your lifetime, even if you are Tibetan you cannot have these visions; thus the visions are not related to the culture, but to a specific spiritual path, knowledge, and transmission. Therefore if people are interested it is important that they deepen their learning and knowledge at which point possibilities can arise. Only realizing the idea of reading a book does not help much. In our lifetime, that is, during the Kyeshi Bardo, many opportunities of learning and preparing ourselves for death can be found.

One day we will arrive at the moment called the Bardo of the Moment of Death. This is another *bardo*, but it does not last long. When we reach this state, the functions of our elements and of our senses slowly dissolve internally. You remember that when we go to bed we relax and then slowly fall asleep: everything dissolves internally with no more thinking, no more seeing, and so forth. We call this process "falling asleep." Of course, death is not like sleeping in this simple way: it is much more difficult. Each function of the elements as well as the functions of the senses dissolves internally and we can have many feelings and fears. How long we have a continuation of this period – called the Bardo of the Moment of Death – depends on the individual, whether during life some preparation was made or not and whether this knowledge was gained or not.

When we fall asleep, for example, we do not dream immediately: sometimes we have no dreams for a long time, sometimes after only a short time. Mostly, dreams arise a short time after falling asleep. Starting to dream means that our mind awakens again. From when we fall asleep until the moment we start to dream, mind does not function. The awakening of mind is associated with the functioning of all the senses, also called the consciousness of the senses in Buddhism and Tantrism, although consciousness is not what is really meant: consciousness is mind; mind is judging and thinking. The senses function without judgment, only absorbing information and communicating it to the mind. So the function of the mental body is associated with mind. In that moment we can have various types of dreams.

In general we have the dreams called karmic dreams, meaning dreams connected with our tensions. If in our lifetime we have experienced serious tensions, we can have this kind of dream even if our sleep is profound. Sometimes we also have dreams connected with past lives: we dream of places, people, or situations that always repeat in the same way, although they never manifested in this life. All these are karmic dreams. Usually people are busy and work hard in the daytime so when they go to bed they immediately sleeps deeply. When sleep is deep we cannot have the special dreams related to our clarity. Most dreams for the majority of people are connected with tension. If we are practitioners and follow a spiritual path, slowly these kinds of dreams diminish and dreams of clarity develop.

Generally, we have dreams of clarity in the early morning. This means that we have already slept for some hours in a heavy sleep so that our sleep becomes lighter and lighter, permitting in that moment more dreams of clarity. A characteristic of dreams of clarity is that they are not connected with our tensions. In particular those dreams are related more to the present situation, but can also regard the future although linked to activities already planned. These are characteristics of the dream of clarity, which are important for practitioners on a spiritual path and also increase the capacity of clarity in daily life because in daily life in the daytime we are totally dependent on the sense organs. In dreams we are not dependent on sense organs and that is why it is said that then we have seven times more clarity. For that reason in a dream we can also do many things such as learn, develop knowledge, and so forth. If we have that capacity and knowledge, there is no difference when we die. All becomes easy in our state of the *bardo* because we are aware of the state that we are in.

In general, when we reach the moment of death and die, if we do not have a spiritual path and some knowledge and understanding of all that is explained in *The Tibetan Book of the Dead*, the manifestations, visions, and so forth will not appear to us and after a little while we will enter the Bardo of Existence. This is similar to entering the dream state when we sleep. When we are in the dream state, we are not aware. Do you know what awareness of dreams means? It means that while you are dreaming you know that you are dreaming. Even if it is a fantastic dream you like very much, you know that it is a dream. When you are aware of dreams and you have a terrible dream, you know that it is only a dream and are not worried. This is called having awareness in dreams. When you do not possess this capacity, the dream is just like the daytime: when you have a nice experience you are happy; if there are problems you are upset. Sometimes you can have a pleasant dream, like winning a big lottery. Then you are overjoyed and try to remember where your ticket is. When you search for it maybe you do not find it and you become worried and upset. When you find it, your joy is doubled: first, you won; second, you found your ticket. You are very happy, but after a little while you wake up and say to yourself, "Oh, how unfortunate. That was only a dream." You see, this is ordinary life and the *bardo* also can be experienced that way. So awareness in dreams is highly important. If you are really aware in dreams and have that experience in your life, when you die you can have awareness in the state of the *bardo* and help yourself greatly. For example, having learned many things in your lifetime, now you can use them. This is called the Bardo of Existence.

When we die we are not immediately in the Bardo of Existence: a passage, a space, exists between death and the Bardo of Existence. If you were a practitioner in your life and learned something, gaining the possibility of being continuously present, this space becomes useful: when you are in the Bardo of Existence you are able to be in the state, in the continuity of presence. This passage or space that manifests after the Bardo of the Moment of Death is called the Bardo of the Dharmata in the Buddhist tradition. Also in *The Tibetan Book of the Dead* it is explained that way.

What does *dharmata* mean? *Dharma* is a Sanskrit word – we use Sanskrit a great deal in the teaching – meaning all phenomena, that is to say, all existence. Sometimes also the teaching of Buddha Shakyamuni is called Dharma. Why? Because all of existence, all of phenomena means infinite things. If we want to know about these infinite things, we need so many lives and even if we studied for many lives we could never finish. For that reason when we receive the teaching of the Buddha, it is said that when we discover one we discover all. That means we are not going to learn about different kinds of outer matters, but knowing that everything outside is in the individual and relates first to the mind, instead of discovering what is external we discover the condition of our own mind. This is the teaching of the Buddha, how he taught. When we discover that, we can understand all phenomena because they are related to our mind. For that reason the teaching of Buddha is called the Dharma.

Dharmata means the real condition of the individual. We have body, energy, and mind: these three are the existence of the individual. The essence of the body and energy and the most important is mind. Some people ask, "What is mind? How is the mind?" It is very easy: when you ask yourself what is mind, this is the mind that is thinking, the mind that is judging. Even if you cannot see or touch it, you can understand that you are thinking. So this is mind. When we know that mind exists, of course we can think also the nature of mind exists because everything has its own nature. Then we ask, "What is the nature of mind?" The nature of mind is called *dharmata* in the ancient Indian language. *Dharmata* means the real nature of our mind. Even if we do not know what the nature of our mind is, at least we can have that idea.

The Bardo of the Dharmata corresponds to the space that extends from death until the mind awakens. When ordinary people die, this space is dark and has no function, but if someone has followed a spiritual path like the one taught in *The Tibetan Book of the Dead* then one understands that even if we fall asleep all the functions of energy are associated. Now that function of energy is passing and in this space there is a kind of presence. In the teaching of *The Tibetan Book of the Dead* this space is called natural light. Natural light does not mean we are doing a kind of visualization or concentrating on and developing something, but rather through the teaching we are discovering that light. Having knowledge of the natural light means that in our lifetime we have received this method or practice of manifestation and also did the visualization of the mandala of the wrathful and peaceful deities. That transmission is part of our nature and our energy and of course in that moment it manifests. When the natural light manifests, people who are in that dimension recognize it and become part of that state: that is the real nature of the individual and those people can have what is called realization. For them the Bardo of Existence will not exist. This is connected only with practitioners. Practitioners who go a little more into detail can find many explanations such as how to develop the four kinds of lights. This has nothing to do with ordinary people who are not practitioners.

For ordinary people in the *bardo* it is very important to recognize that they are in that state. If they had some contact with this teaching of *The Tibetan Book of the Dead*, they also have a connection, and some communication is then possible. For example, someone is dying. In the moment of death we communicate with that person, saying, "Now you are dying, do not worry, do not create attachment because it will not help you. More important is that you notice that you are now dying; this is normal for everybody, everybody must die. Now this moment is arriving for you: try to be present, and when you are in the state of the Bardo of Existence remember what you received in your lifetime, such as information about the *Bardo Thödrol*." Thus we try to help the person remember, and we introduce knowledge in this way.

Three days after death we do a kind of introduction because usually it takes more or less three days for the dead person to emerge in the state of the Bardo of Existence. Once they are there we communicate with them, saying, for example, "Now do not worry; you have died; you no longer have a body." Most people do not understand that they are dead because of strong attachment to life and to all of existence and in particular to their physical body. Therefore, even if dead, they feel that they are still human.

You continue, saying, "When you stand in the light you have no shadow; when you wish to go outside you need not go through the door, you can go through the wall. This means you have no physical body." Thus different introductions and reasoning can help the dead person understand. So they more or less come to understand that they are dead and this is important because otherwise they can never overcome their attachment and continuously create many problems. When they know that they are dead, they do their best. Also good practitioners with capacity can communicate with them and make understood that the dead should do what they learned in their practice during their lifetime, and so forth. In that way we can help.

Particularly in Tibet, in the traditional way and also according to *The Tibetan Book of the Dead,* when someone dies *pujas* and practice are done for him or her for forty-nine days, that is, seven weeks. From the time of death, each seven days an explanation is given of another kind of death. Of course the physical body does not exist. The dead person may not really feel dead, but a process occurs through which slowly attachment diminishes and the discovery emerges more and more that he or she is in the state of the *bardo*. We do the introduction for the first time on the third day. If it does not succeed then we introduce again seven days after the death. This is because there is another process of death and in that moment that person has a little more clarity. Even if we do not succeed precisely in our explanation, we do it again after seven more days, and we proceed like that for forty-nine days. Forty-nine days is considered the approximate duration of the *bardo* for most people, although it does not mean that the length of the *bardo* is really limited in that way. Some beings remain in the *bardo* for a very long time, others only a short time like one or two weeks.

Everybody has his or her own karma. Karma means the potentiality of actions. Some people think that karma is a philosophical concept of Eastern countries. Karma is not really a philosophy of the East. It is a Sanskrit term that means action, some way we have acted. Our actions can be good or bad or neutral. If we act in a good way such as performing good actions, this will produce positive consequences. If we do something negative, of course the consequences will be negative. This is not only an Eastern belief, but also a Western and global one. In a film that shows a bad person, for example, the person who is performing negative actions at the end finishes badly. This is karma, or you can also call it action. In any case karma produces the potentiality of good or bad. When we have accumulated many good or bad actions, we experience the *bardo* state according to the potentiality of these karmas. Practitioners who have realized something, who have real knowledge and are free in their condition are not dependent on karma. Otherwise we are always dependent on karma.

For example, in our life sometimes we have many problems. These indicate the maturation of our negative karma as for example, we contract illnesses. Sometimes we have illnesses related mainly to the physical level and those are much easier to cure with medicine. Sometimes our illness is related more to the energy level; then it is a little more complicated, because unlike a physical disturbance, we cannot see or touch energy. For example, if our energy is unbalanced, then of course we will have many problems, illnesses, and also in ordinary life everything will go badly. When our energy is disordered and its function or the function of the five elements is damaged, we do not have sufficient protective energy. In this case, if negativities exist within our circumstances, we will be the first to receive them. Still more difficult is if the problem is connected to our mind. Mental problems cannot be cured only with medicines. This is how our body, energy level, and mind are related.

Trying to cure illnesses, for example, we can easily receive many negative provocations if our protective energy is not sufficient. Negative provocation conditions also exist in our dimension, for example, related to our energy level, to the five elements, or whatever we are dealing with in our lifetime. Still worse, we can receive attacks of something like black magic. These are what are called negative provocations. Today we have so many illnesses like cancer and AIDS. These illnesses not only exist on physical or energy levels, but can also be combined with negative provocations. This negative energy must be controlled; otherwise there is no possibility of cure. In Tibetan medicine we can cure with mantras and such practices. With these kinds of illnesses, when we cure in this way to control negative energy, the medicines and other therapies will function in a perfect way. Sometimes, even if we cure with mantras and so forth, we have no one hundred percent guarantee that we can cure everything. Why? Because many of these illnesses are connected with our karma. When we have acted in an extremely negative way and our karma is maturing in this moment, we can be paying for that with these illnesses. For purifying the negative potentiality of this karma we need time and cannot purify that easily. When we have these kinds of illnesses we also do not have much time to try to cure ourselves. That is an example of why it is important to know that karma is connected to our condition.

A metaphor for our existence in the Bardo of Existence is that our state is like a feather drifting in space. The feather is not free to decide to go here or there; it is dependent on the direction of the wind. The wind is an example of the potentiality of karma. Because of that condition we can have different kinds of rebirth in different dimensions. For overcoming this problem we can do many things and *The Tibetan Book of the Dead* contains rich explanations. I cannot explain everything here. I am just giving a little advice. If you are interested, you can read and study many versions of the *Tibetan Book of the Dead*. It is important that you know that something can be done in this life, because our life is short. People always think they still have many years, but nobody knows. We have no guarantee. Some think that way because they are very young, but young or old, there is not much difference. Our life is like a lit candle in an open place: there are so many secondary causes, that can eliminate our life, like the wind. It is important not only to look at what is before us, but to understand the nature of our existence and to continue that way. Everybody should do his or her best. *The Tibetan Book of the Dead* is very useful in that regard. If you are interested you should investigate this knowledge a little deeper. It is not only a history or an intellectual study: it is something concretely related to our existence. So do your best. Now, if you have questions I can reply.

Q: Since the central point in the *bardo* and in life is acquiring knowledge, and since you invite us to read *The Tibetan Book of the Dead* because it helps us live our life, could you also tell us in what way we should read it?

A: For reading the *Bardo Thödrol* you need to receive the transmission of that teaching; otherwise only reading it does not work. The *Bardo Thödrol* contains explanations of how the *bardo* is, but if you want to apply them, you need to learn the instructions. When you have learned the instructions, you know how to do something. If you do not wish to read the book, if you just want some enjoyment and are satisfied with knowing a little, you can watch films of it that have been made and can have a global idea.

Q: If a person who is not a practitioner dies is there any way to help him make undergoing the death process easier?

A: If they are not practitioners and are just interested in listening, of course there is some benefit, but they cannot really enter in that knowledge.

Q: When the dying person is not feeling anything anymore, in one chapter it is said there is a sort of light. Can you help the person in that moment?

A: For helping some communication needs to exist with that person. If there is no communication we cannot help. For having communication that person must be present, even if dead. Even so, there is a kind of presence or communication.

Q: In the book it is said that when the person has died you have to leave the body without touching it for three days. In the Western world this is not possible because you have to bury or burn the body immediately. How can you help in that case?

A: The most important thing is that doctors check that the person is really dead. I once heard that somebody who was already in the cemetery awoke. [laughter]

Q: I would like to know if time has the same meaning when one is dead as when a person is alive.

A: Our consideration of time, day and night and so forth, is our dualistic vision. In death we cannot calibrate time as we do in life.

Q: I have a spiritual commitment to recite mantras every night to Guru Padmasambhava for dead people. Is there a connection between me and the Guru because of that?

A: If you have a connection with the transmission and teaching, of course there is.

Q: Is death connected to reincarnation? Is it a continuous process? Just after death is there reincarnation or what is the relation between death and reincarnation?

A: You mean rebirth? Rebirth always exists because we are living in time. The immediacy of a rebirth is connected to karma. If you are a realized person, then you are free. Otherwise, as I already said, everything depends on karma. Forty-nine days is generally considered the length of the bardo, but there is no limitation of time. I said this already.

Professor Alfonso M. García Hernández:

We want to thank again Master Chögyal Namkhai Norbu and the International Dzogchen Community and congratulate them on this event and for the Third Tibetan Cultural Week, which we hope will continue in the future because of the great interest created.

1